FITNESS FOR HEALTH

FITNESS FOR HEALTH

TIM KORSA

CONTENTS

FITNESS FOR HEALTH — vii
TEXT INSERT — viii

1. Introduction to Fitness & Health — 1
2. Understanding Your Body — 8
3. Types of Sports and Their Benefits — 16
4. Building a Fitness Routine — 40
5. Strength Training for Everyone — 47
6. Cardio for Health & Fat Loss — 56
7. Nutrition for Sports Performance — 73
8. Mental Benefits of Sports — 85
9. Injury Prevention & Healing — 94
10. Staying Motivated Long-Term — 110
11. How Fitness Helps you overcome Depression — 125
12. Special Training for Different Ages — 133
13. Conclusion: Living the Strong Life — 153

CHAPTER — 157
TEXT INSERT — 158
ABOUT THE AUTHOR — 159

FITNESS FOR HEALTH

Copyright © 2025 by TIM KORSA

All rights reserved. No part of this book may be reproduced in any manner whatsoever without written permission except in the case of brief quotations embodied in critical articles and reviews.

ISBN-13: 9798901488515

First Printing, 2025

Introduction to Fitness & Health

Chapter 1

Introduction to Fitness & Health

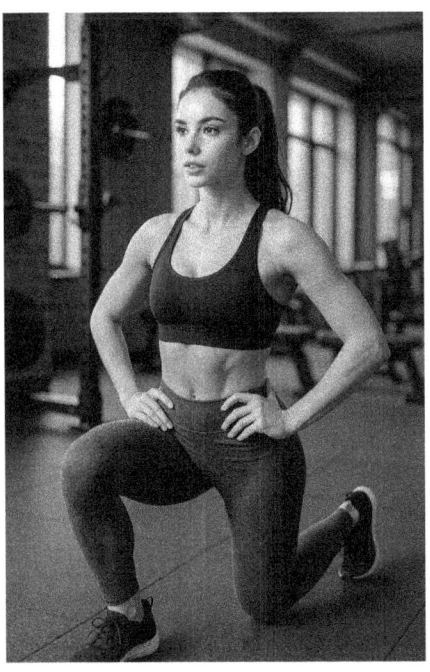

1. Why Fitness Matters

Fitness is one of the most important foundations of a healthy and successful life. It affects every major system in the body and determines how well you move, feel, think, and age. Regular physical activity strengthens the heart, lungs, muscles, and bones while improving mental health and emotional well-being. Fitness is not only about looking better — it is essential for long-term health, daily energy, and overall quality of life.

Physical activity strengthens the **heart**, helping it pump blood more efficiently and reducing the risk of heart disease, high blood pressure, and stroke. A stronger heart delivers more oxygen and nutrients throughout the body, improving endurance and helping you perform daily tasks with less fatigue. At the same time, fitness enhances **lung capacity**, allowing you to breathe deeper and more efficiently. Better oxygen delivery increases overall stamina and supports healthier cells and organs.

Regular exercise builds and protects **muscles** and **bones**, keeping the body strong and stable. Strong muscles support joints, reduce the risk of injuries, and improve posture. Weight-bearing exercises increase **bone density**, which is crucial for preventing osteoporosis and fractures, especially as we age. Fitness also boosts the **immune system**, helping the body fight illness more effectively and recover faster.

One of the most visible benefits of fitness is **weight control**. Exercise burns calories, increases metabolism, and improves the body's ability to use energy. This helps reduce body fat, regulate blood sugar, and lower the risk of conditions such as diabetes. Beyond physical changes, fitness plays a huge role in **mental health**. Exercise triggers the release of endorphins — natural chemicals that reduce stress, improve mood, increase confidence, and help manage anxiety and depression.

Ultimately, fitness improves **longevity**, extending both the length and the quality of your life. Regular physical activity lowers the risk of chronic disease, strengthens the body's systems, and promotes better sleep, mobility, and independence. Fitness makes everyday life easier —

walking, climbing stairs, lifting objects, working, and even relaxing all become more comfortable when the body is healthy and strong.

In simple terms, fitness matters because it makes you feel better, look better, and live better. It is one of the most powerful investments you can make in your body, your mind, and your future.

2. How Sports Improve the Body

Sports are one of the most effective ways to strengthen and transform the body. When you participate in physical activities such as running, swimming, cycling, martial arts, or team sports, the entire body works together — heart, lungs, muscles, bones, and nervous system. This full-body engagement makes sports far more dynamic than simple exercise and delivers powerful health benefits that improve how the body performs, feels, and ages.

Sports strengthen the **cardiovascular system**, which includes the heart and blood vessels. When you play sports that involve movement, speed, and endurance, your heart pumps faster and becomes stronger. Over time, this improves circulation, lowers blood pressure, increases oxygen delivery, and reduces the risk of heart disease. A well-trained heart is more efficient and healthier, making everyday tasks easier.

Sports also improve **lung function** by increasing the body's demand for oxygen. Activities such as running, basketball, or swimming require controlled breathing and deeper inhales, which expand lung capacity. Stronger lungs supply more oxygen to the muscles and brain, boosting stamina and endurance. This allows you to move longer, recover faster, and feel less tired throughout the day.

One of the most obvious benefits of sports is the development of **muscles**. Different sports activate different muscle groups — sprinting builds powerful legs, swimming strengthens the upper body, martial arts develop core stability, and soccer enhances agility. Sports also improve muscle coordination, reaction time, and balance. Strong, well-trained muscles protect the joints, reduce injury risk, and support better posture.

Sports also have a major impact on **bone health**. Jumping, running, and weight-bearing movements stimulate bone growth and increase bone density. This strengthens the skeletal system and lowers the risk of fractures and osteoporosis later in life. The combination of strong muscles and strong bones forms the physical foundation of a healthy body.

Another key benefit is improved **metabolism**. Sports increase calorie burning, improve insulin sensitivity, and help regulate body fat levels. A more active metabolism supports better weight control and reduces the risk of diabetes and metabolic disorders.

Playing sports also trains the **nervous system**. Quick movements, strategic decisions, hand-eye coordination, and balance all sharpen the brain-body connection. This enhances reflexes, agility, focus, and overall athletic performance.

In short, sports improve the body by strengthening the heart, lungs, muscles, bones, metabolism, and nervous system. They build power, endurance, coordination, and resilience. Regular participation in sports not only enhances physical performance but also supports long-term health, creating a healthier and more capable body for life.

3. How Sports Improve the Mind

Sports do far more than strengthen the body — they also improve the mind. Physical activity has a powerful influence on mental clarity, emotional stability, confidence, and cognitive function. When you engage in sports regularly, your brain receives more oxygen, releases beneficial chemicals, and becomes better at managing stress, decision-making, and focus. The mental benefits are so significant that many experts consider sports one of the most effective natural tools for improving mental health and brain performance.

One of the most important ways sports improve the mind is through the release of **endorphins**, often called "feel-good chemicals." Endorphins reduce stress, elevate mood, and create a sense of well-being. This is why people often feel happier and more relaxed after physical activity. Sports also lower levels of cortisol, the body's stress hormone, helping reduce anxiety and emotional tension.

Sports enhance **cognitive function**, which includes your ability to think clearly, learn quickly, and remember information. When you move your body, blood flow to the brain increases, delivering more oxygen and nutrients. This supports the growth of new brain cells, improves neural connections, and strengthens areas responsible for memory, concentration, and problem-solving. Research consistently shows that people who stay physically active have better focus and slower cognitive decline as they age.

Another major benefit is improved **discipline and self-control**. Sports require consistency, practice, patience, and commitment. These habits build mental toughness and teach the brain how to push through challenges. Athletes learn how to set goals, stay motivated, manage failure, and develop a strong mindset that carries into all areas of life — work, relationships, and personal growth.

Sports also provide powerful **emotional benefits**. Participating in physical activity helps reduce symptoms of depression and anxiety by balancing hormones and providing a productive outlet for frustration or negative thoughts. Many people experience improved sleep patterns from regular activity, which further supports emotional stability and sharper thinking.

Beyond individual benefits, sports strengthen the mind through **social interaction**. Team sports teach communication, cooperation, and trust. Being part of a group gives a sense of belonging and builds confidence. Even solo sports, such as running or swimming, help individuals feel connected through shared goals or training communities.

In summary, sports improve the mind by reducing stress, boosting mood, sharpening focus, strengthening memory, and increasing confidence. They build discipline, emotional resilience, and mental clarity. By improving the brain's chemistry, structure, and performance, sports create a stronger, healthier, and more positive mindset that supports every area of life.

4. Common Myths About Exercise

Despite how important fitness is, many people are held back by misinformation and outdated beliefs. These common myths often create confusion, fear, or unrealistic expectations — stopping people from starting or sticking to an exercise routine. Understanding the truth behind these myths helps you train safely, effectively, and confidently.

One of the most widespread myths is **"You need to exercise for hours every day to get results."** In reality, even 20–30 minutes of moderate activity can significantly improve health. Short, consistent workouts are far more effective than long, inconsistent ones. Your body responds to regular movement, not extreme sessions.

Another myth is **"Cardio alone is enough for good health."** While cardio is great for the heart and lungs, it cannot replace strength training. Building muscle improves metabolism, supports joints, strengthens bones, and helps prevent injury. A balanced routine includes strength, cardio, and flexibility work — not just one type.

Many people also believe **"Lifting weights makes you bulky."** This is incorrect. Building large muscle mass requires very specific training, high-calorie diets, and genetics. Regular strength training actually tones the body, increases metabolism, and improves functional strength without adding excessive size. For most people, weights help them look leaner, not bigger.

A common excuse is **"I'm too old to start exercising."** Fitness benefits every age group. Elderly adults can improve balance, mobility, heart health, and independence through safe, low-impact exercises. The human body is designed to move, and it responds positively at every stage of life. It's never too late to start.

Another damaging myth is **"Pain equals progress."** While some discomfort is normal when the body adapts, sharp pain or joint pain is a warning sign. Good workouts challenge the body, but they do not injure it. Proper form, recovery, and listening to your body are essential for safe progress.

Many also think **"You must be in shape before joining a gym or playing a sport."** The truth is the opposite: gyms, sports, and trainers exist to help people get in shape. Everyone starts somewhere, and no one is expected to be perfect from the beginning. Progress comes from practice, not perfection.

Finally, some people believe **"If you stop exercising, your muscles turn into fat."** Muscle and fat are two different tissues — one cannot transform into the other. If you stop training, muscles shrink and you may gain fat due to reduced activity, but they do not convert into one another.

In summary, common exercise myths often create unnecessary fear or confusion. Understanding the truth — that fitness is flexible, accessible, and beneficial for every age and body — empowers you to build a healthy routine that works for you. Breaking these myths helps you train smarter, safer, and with greater confidence.

2

Understanding Your Body

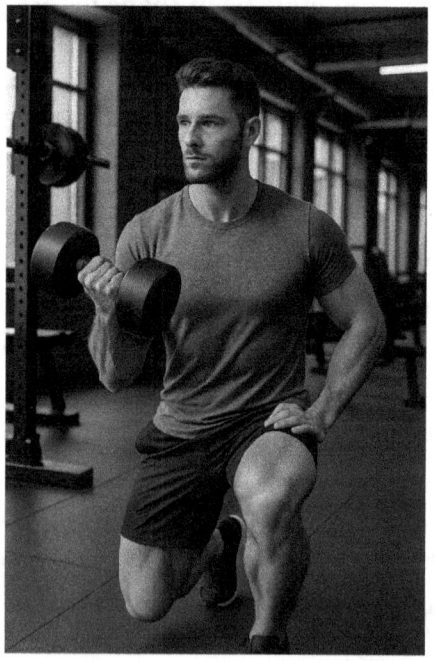

1. Major Muscle Groups

The major muscle groups of the body form the foundation for all movement, strength, stability, and physical health. Each group plays a unique role, but they work together as a coordinated system that allows you to walk, lift, breathe, jump, run, and maintain proper posture. Understanding why these muscle groups are important helps you train smarter and support a healthier, stronger body.

The **deltoids, pectorals, biceps, triceps, and upper-body muscles** are responsible for pushing, pulling, lifting, and stabilizing your shoulders and arms. These muscles support daily tasks such as carrying groceries, lifting objects, and reaching overhead. Strengthening these areas helps prevent shoulder injuries and improves posture.

The **core muscles**, including the rectus abdominis, obliques, and lower-back muscles, are crucial for stability. The core acts like the body's foundation, supporting every movement you make. A strong core improves balance, reduces back pain, protects the spine, and enhances athletic performance in every sport. Without a strong core, even simple movements become harder and more risky.

The **back muscles**, such as the latissimus dorsi and trapezius, help maintain posture, support the spine, and create pulling strength. A strong back keeps the body aligned, reduces strain on the lower back, and prevents slouching. These muscles are essential for lifting, carrying, and rotating the body safely.

The **legs contain some of the largest muscle groups** in the body — the quadriceps, hamstrings, glutes, calves, and hip adductors. These muscles are responsible for walking, running, jumping, climbing, and maintaining balance. Strong legs improve mobility, increase power, and support joint health. They are also critical for preventing injuries in the knees and hips.

The **glutes** (buttocks muscles) are among the most powerful muscles in the body. They stabilize the pelvis, protect the lower back, and produce force for walking, sprinting, and lifting. Weak glutes contribute to back pain, poor posture, and decreased athletic performance.

Even the **smaller muscle groups** — such as the calves, forearms, and tibialis anterior — play important roles in balance, grip strength, and stabilizing your movements. These muscles allow you to walk safely, absorb impact, and perform precise actions with your hands.

Training all major muscle groups keeps the body balanced. If one group is weak, other muscles overwork to compensate, increasing the risk of injury. Balanced strength improves posture, boosts metabolism, increases energy levels, and enhances performance in sports and daily life.

In summary, the major muscle groups are important because they support movement, protect joints, stabilize the body, prevent injuries, and maintain overall strength and mobility. A healthy, balanced muscular system allows you to live an active, pain-free, and independent life.

2. Cardiovascular System

The cardiovascular system is one of the most vital systems in the human body. It is responsible for delivering oxygen, nutrients, and hormones to every cell while removing waste products such as carbon dioxide. This system includes the **heart, blood vessels**, and **blood**, working together in a continuous cycle that keeps you alive, energized, and healthy. When your cardiovascular system is strong, your entire body performs better — physically, mentally, and emotionally.

At the center of the system is the **heart**, a powerful muscular pump that beats about 60–100 times per minute. Each heartbeat pushes blood through a vast network of blood vessels. **Arteries** carry oxygen-rich blood from the heart to the organs and muscles. **Veins** return oxygen-depleted blood back to the heart, where it is sent to the lungs to be refilled with oxygen. This constant circulation provides the energy your body needs to move, think, heal, and function.

The cardiovascular system also regulates **blood pressure**, which is the force of blood pushing against the walls of your arteries. Healthy blood pressure ensures that the heart and vessels are not overstressed. When blood pressure is too high, the heart works harder, increasing the risk of heart disease and stroke. When it is too low, you may feel fatigued, dizzy, or weak. Keeping the cardiovascular system healthy helps maintain stable, efficient circulation.

A well-functioning cardiovascular system improves **oxygen delivery**. Every cell in the body needs oxygen to produce energy. When you exercise, your muscles demand more oxygen, causing your heart to pump faster and your lungs to work harder. Over time, this training strengthens your heart, allowing it to pump more blood with less effort. This results in better stamina, faster recovery, and more energy throughout the day.

The cardiovascular system also plays a key role in **temperature control**, transporting heat generated in the muscles to the skin, where it can be released. This helps prevent overheating and allows the body to stay cool during physical activity.

A healthy cardiovascular system has major long-term effects on your life. Strong circulation supports brain health, improving memory, focus, and mental clarity. It reduces the risk of chronic diseases such as hypertension, diabetes, and heart attacks. It boosts endurance, enabling you to perform daily activities with ease — from walking and climbing stairs to playing sports and enjoying outdoor activities.

On the other hand, a weak cardiovascular system leads to fatigue, low energy, poor endurance, and higher risk of disease. Lifestyle factors such as lack of exercise, smoking, stress, and poor diet can damage blood vessels and weaken the heart.

In summary, the cardiovascular system works as the body's engine — constantly delivering oxygen, fuel, and nutrients while supporting every organ. When kept strong through regular exercise, healthy eating, and good habits, it greatly improves quality of life, longevity, and overall well-being.

3. Respiratory System

The respiratory system is the body's essential life-support system that provides oxygen — the fuel every cell needs to survive. It is responsible for taking in oxygen from the air, delivering it to the bloodstream, and removing carbon dioxide, a waste product created by your cells.

Without a healthy respiratory system, the body cannot produce energy, your organs cannot function properly, and life cannot be sustained.

The process begins with **breathing**, or ventilation. When you inhale, air enters through the nose or mouth, travels down the trachea, and moves into two large tubes called the bronchi. These bronchi branch into smaller tubes inside the lungs, ending in millions of tiny air sacs called **alveoli**. The alveoli are surrounded by capillaries — tiny blood vessels where gas exchange happens. Oxygen from the air passes through the thin walls of the alveoli into the blood, while carbon dioxide from the blood passes out into the lungs to be exhaled. This exchange happens every second of the day, even while you sleep.

Once oxygen enters the bloodstream, the **cardiovascular system** carries it throughout the body. Your organs, muscles, brain, and tissues use oxygen to produce energy through a process called cellular respiration. When oxygen levels are low, the body becomes tired, weak, and unable to perform properly. This is why strong lung function is essential for physical performance and overall health.

The respiratory system also plays a major role in **regulating the body's pH balance**, helping maintain the correct internal environment for vital processes. By controlling the amount of carbon dioxide you exhale, your lungs help keep your blood from becoming too acidic or too alkaline.

Physical activity strengthens the respiratory system by training the lungs and diaphragm to work more efficiently. When you exercise, your breathing rate increases, forcing your lungs to expand more fully and deliver more oxygen. Over time, this improves lung capacity, increases oxygen delivery, and enhances stamina. A stronger respiratory system improves performance in sports, daily tasks, and overall energy levels.

The respiratory system also supports the **immune system**. The nose filters dust, bacteria, and viruses through tiny hairs and mucus. Coughing and sneezing are protective reflexes that clear harmful particles. Healthy lungs provide strong defense against respiratory illnesses such as flu, pneumonia, asthma complications, and infections.

If the respiratory system becomes weakened by smoking, pollution, inactivity, or diseases, the body struggles to get enough oxygen. This can lead to fatigue, shortness of breath, low energy, and serious health conditions. Protecting your lungs through fitness, clean air, and healthy habits is essential for long-term well-being.

In summary, the respiratory system is vital because it supplies oxygen, removes waste, supports energy production, helps regulate body functions, and protects against illness. Strong lungs and efficient breathing are key to living a healthy, active, and energetic life.

4. How Energy & Metabolism Work

Energy and metabolism are at the core of how the human body functions. Every movement you make — walking, breathing, thinking, digesting, exercising, even sleeping — requires energy. Metabolism is the process your body uses to convert the food you eat into usable energy. Understanding how energy and metabolism work helps you improve your health, manage weight, boost performance, and increase overall vitality.

The process begins with **food intake**. Everything you eat contains nutrients such as carbohydrates, proteins, and fats. During digestion, the body breaks these nutrients down into smaller molecules:

- **Carbohydrates** become glucose (sugar),
- **Fats** become fatty acids, and
- **Proteins** become amino acids.

These molecules enter the bloodstream and are transported to cells throughout the body. Inside each cell, structures called **mitochondria** convert these nutrients into energy through a biochemical process known as **cellular respiration**. This energy is stored in molecules called

ATP (adenosine triphosphate). ATP is the body's "energy currency" — the fuel your cells use for every task.

Metabolism includes two major parts:

1. **Catabolism** — the breakdown of molecules to release energy.
2. **Anabolism** — the building or repairing of tissues, such as muscle growth.

These two processes work together to keep your body alive, healthy, and functional.

Your **metabolic rate** is the speed at which your body uses energy. Even when resting, the body burns calories to keep essential systems running — heart pumping, lungs breathing, brain functioning, and body temperature regulated. This is known as **basal metabolic rate (BMR)**. The more lean muscle mass you have, the higher your metabolism, because muscle tissue requires more energy than fat tissue.

Physical activity significantly increases energy use. During exercise, your muscles require more oxygen and nutrients to produce ATP quickly. This speeds up metabolism both during and after the workout — a phenomenon called **EPOC (excess post-exercise oxygen consumption)**, or the "afterburn effect." This is why regular exercise helps with fat loss and improves overall energy levels.

Hormones also play a major role in metabolism. Hormones such as insulin, thyroid hormones, cortisol, and adrenaline regulate how fast or slow the body converts food into energy. When these hormones are out of balance, metabolism may slow down, causing fatigue, weight gain, or difficulty building muscle.

Energy and metabolism affect every part of life. A strong, efficient metabolism gives you more vitality, better endurance, improved brain function, and stable weight. On the other hand, a slow or disrupted metabolism leads to low energy, poor focus, weight gain, and decreased performance.

In summary, energy and metabolism work together to power every function in the body. By eating nutritious foods, staying active, building muscle, and maintaining healthy habits, you support a strong metabolism that keeps your body energized, balanced, and performing at its best.

3
Types of Sports and Their Benefits

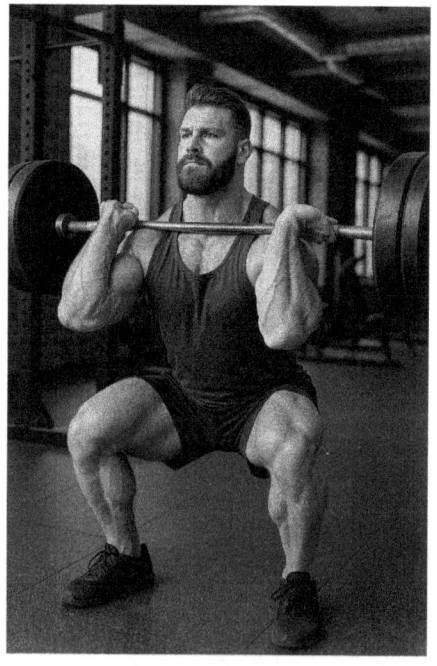

Strength sports like **weightlifting** and **wrestling** are some of the most physically demanding and rewarding activities. They develop power, discipline, and confidence, but they also come with challenges that require responsibility, proper technique, and smart training.

◈ Benefits (PLUS)

1. Builds Powerful Muscles and Strength
Strength sports activate nearly all major muscle groups.
Weightlifting increases muscle mass, bone density, power, and explosive strength, while wrestling builds full-body functional strength and conditioning.

2. Strengthens Bones and Joints
Heavy lifting and wrestling place controlled stress on the bones.
This stimulates bone growth and increases density, helping prevent osteoporosis and fractures later in life.

3. Boosts Metabolism
More muscle equals a faster metabolism.
Strength athletes burn more calories even at rest, which helps with long-term weight control and body-fat reduction.

4. Improves Discipline and Mental Toughness
Both sports demand focus, patience, and resilience.
Athletes learn how to set goals, overcome challenges, and push through mental barriers — skills that carry into everyday life.

5. Enhances Athletic Performance
Strength training improves speed, stability, balance, and coordination.
Wrestling increases agility, reflexes, and endurance, making athletes better in many other sports.

6. Increases Confidence
Achieving strength goals, mastering techniques, and improving physical ability boosts self-esteem and mental strength.

7. Excellent for Full-Body Conditioning

Weightlifting builds power.
Wrestling builds power, cardio, flexibility, and durability.
Together they create one of the best full-body fitness combinations.

◈ Drawbacks (MINUS)

1. Higher Risk of Injury if Done Incorrectly

Poor form, excessive weight, or lack of proper warm-up can cause:

- Muscle strains
- Joint injuries
- Sprains
- Lower-back issues
  In wrestling, impact and resistance against an opponent increase risk if technique is poor.

2. Requires Proper Coaching and Technique

Strength sports are safe when taught correctly, but beginners often struggle without guidance.
Bad habits can form quickly, leading to setbacks.

3. Physically Demanding Recovery

Heavy strength training stresses the body.
Recovering requires:

- Proper sleep
- Good nutrition
- Rest days
  Without this, progress slows and fatigue rises.

4. Overtraining Risk

Pushing too hard too fast can exhaust the muscles and nervous system.
Wrestlers, in particular, often face intense training schedules that require balance to avoid burnout.

5. Time and Consistency Required

Strength progress takes commitment.
You must train consistently, often multiple times per week, to see results.

6. Wrestling Weight Cuts (if competing)

Some athletes cut weight to reach a lower class.
If done incorrectly, this can affect:

- Hydration
- Energy levels
- Overall health
  Safe nutrition planning is essential.

Summary

Strength sports offer powerful benefits: stronger muscles, higher confidence, better metabolism, improved bone health, and unmatched full-body conditioning. However, they also require discipline, proper technique, patience, and respect for recovery and safety.

When practiced responsibly, **weightlifting and wrestling are among the most rewarding and transformative sports for both body and mind.**

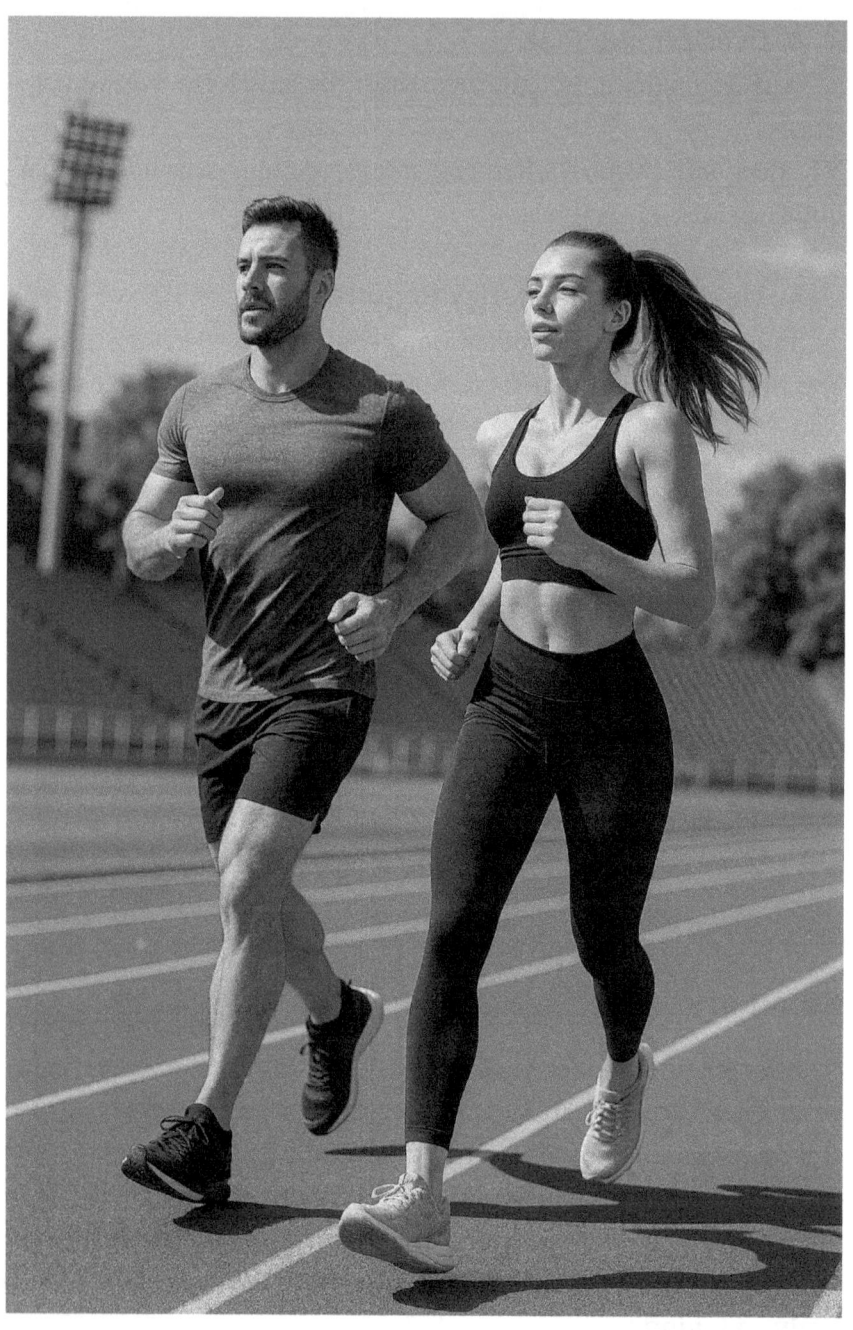

1. **Endurance Sports (Running, Cycling)**

Endurance sports like **running** and **cycling** are two of the most popular forms of exercise worldwide. They strengthen the heart, improve stamina, and boost mental health. However, like all sports, they also come with challenges and risks that should be understood for safe, effective training.

◈ Benefits (PLUS)

1. Excellent for Heart and Lung Health
Running and cycling increase heart rate, strengthen the heart muscle, and improve circulation.
They also enhance lung capacity and oxygen delivery, making the cardiovascular and respiratory systems more efficient.

2. Great for Weight Control and Fat Loss
Endurance sports burn a high number of calories.
Regular training helps reduce body fat, maintain a healthy weight, and improve metabolism — especially when combined with proper nutrition.

3. Builds Strong Stamina and Energy Levels
These sports train the body to use energy more effectively. Over time, you gain:

- Higher endurance
- Better overall energy
- Less fatigue during daily activities

4. Improves Mental Health and Mood

Running and cycling release endorphins, reducing stress, anxiety, and depression.

They provide a sense of freedom, mental clarity, and emotional balance.

5. Low Equipment Requirement (Especially Running)

Running needs nothing but shoes.

Cycling requires a bike but offers smooth, low-impact training.

6. Strengthens Legs and Core

Both sports build strong:

- Quadriceps
- Hamstrings
- Glutes
- Calves
- Hip muscles

Cycling particularly helps individuals who need low-impact leg strength.

7. Great for Longevity

Regular endurance training is associated with:

- Lower risk of heart disease
- Lower blood pressure
- Better cholesterol levels
- Longer lifespan

◈ Drawbacks (MINUS)

1. Risk of Overuse Injuries
Endurance sports involve repetitive motion.
Common problems include:

- Shin splints
- Knee pain
- Plantar fasciitis
- Lower back pain

Cycling can also cause hip tightness and neck strain if posture is poor.

2. High Impact Stress (Running)
Running puts impact pressure on joints.
Without proper footwear or technique, this can lead to joint irritation or long-term discomfort.

3. Time-Consuming
Endurance improvement requires longer sessions.
To see results, you often need 30–60 minutes of activity per day.

4. Weather Dependence
Running and cycling can be difficult in:

- Extreme heat
- Rain
- Snow
- Cold

This may require access to indoor equipment like treadmills or stationary bikes.

5. Can Lead to Muscle Loss if Not Balanced

Excessive endurance training without strength work may cause:

- Muscle breakdown
- Reduced power
- Lower metabolism

A balanced routine is essential.

6. Requires Proper Hydration and Nutrition

Endurance athletes burn a lot of calories and lose electrolytes. Failing to replace them can lead to fatigue, cramps, or dizziness.

Summary

Endurance sports like running and cycling are exceptional for cardiovascular health, weight control, and mental wellness. They build strong legs, high stamina, and long-lasting energy.

However, they also require proper technique, balanced training, and smart recovery to avoid overuse injuries and fatigue.

When done correctly, endurance sports are one of the most effective ways to build a healthy, strong, and resilient body.

2. Team Sports (Soccer, Basketball)

Team sports like **soccer** and **basketball** are among the most popular physical activities worldwide. They offer a powerful combination of physical conditioning, mental development, and social interaction. These sports build athleticism and teamwork, but they also come with challenges that athletes should understand to train safely and effectively.

◈ Benefits (PLUS)

1. Full-Body Conditioning

Soccer and basketball require running, jumping, sprinting, and quick directional changes.
These movements strengthen:

- Legs (quads, hamstrings, glutes, calves)
- Core muscles
- Cardiovascular and respiratory systems
  This creates excellent all-around fitness.

2. Improves Coordination, Agility & Reflexes

Both sports demand fast reaction time and dynamic movement. Players develop:

- Hand-eye coordination
- Footwork skills
- Balance and agility
- Quick decision-making

These skills benefit athletes in everyday life and other sports.

3. Great for Heart Health

Team sports involve continuous motion that elevates heart rate. This improves:

- Circulation
- Cardiac strength
- Lung capacity
- Overall endurance

Regular participation lowers the risk of heart disease.

4. Builds Strong Social Skills & Teamwork

Team sports require communication, cooperation, trust, and shared responsibility.

Players learn how to:

- Work with others
- Handle conflict
- Support teammates
- Lead and follow

These social skills transfer into school, work, and relationships.

5. Boosts Mental Health & Confidence

Playing on a team builds:

- Self-esteem
- A sense of belonging
- Motivation
- Stress relief

Winning, improving skills, and contributing to the team improve overall emotional well-being.

6. Teaches Discipline & Responsibility

Players must practice, show up on time, follow rules, and stay committed.

These habits build discipline that helps in every part of life.

◈ Drawbacks (MINUS)

1. Higher Risk of Injury

Because of fast play, contact, and sudden movements, common injuries include:

- Ankle sprains
- Knee injuries (including ACL tears)
- Muscle strains
- Collisions and falls

Proper warm-up and technique reduce risks.

2. Requires Team Availability

Unlike solo sports, you need teammates, schedules, and often a coach.
This can limit flexibility and make regular training harder.

3. Competitive Pressure

Games and tournaments can create:

- Stress
- Anxiety
- Fear of mistakes
- Performance pressure

For some players, this pressure may reduce enjoyment.

4. Possible Overtraining

League seasons can be demanding with:

- Frequent games
- Intense practices
- Travel
  Without proper rest, players may experience fatigue or burnout.

5. Not Always Beginner-Friendly

New players may feel intimidated by:

- Fast pace
- Skill level differences
- Team expectations

But with time and practice, confidence grows.

6. Requires Equipment & Facilities
While not extremely expensive, players need:

- Balls
- Shoes
- Goals or hoops
- Fields or courts
   Access may be limited depending on location.

Summary

Team sports like soccer and basketball offer incredible physical, mental, and social benefits. They improve endurance, strength, coordination, and confidence while teaching teamwork and discipline. However, they also require safe training, proper recovery, and a supportive environment to avoid injury and burnout.

When balanced correctly, team sports are one of the most enjoyable and complete forms of fitness.

TYPES OF SPORTS AND THEIR BENEFITS — | 29 |

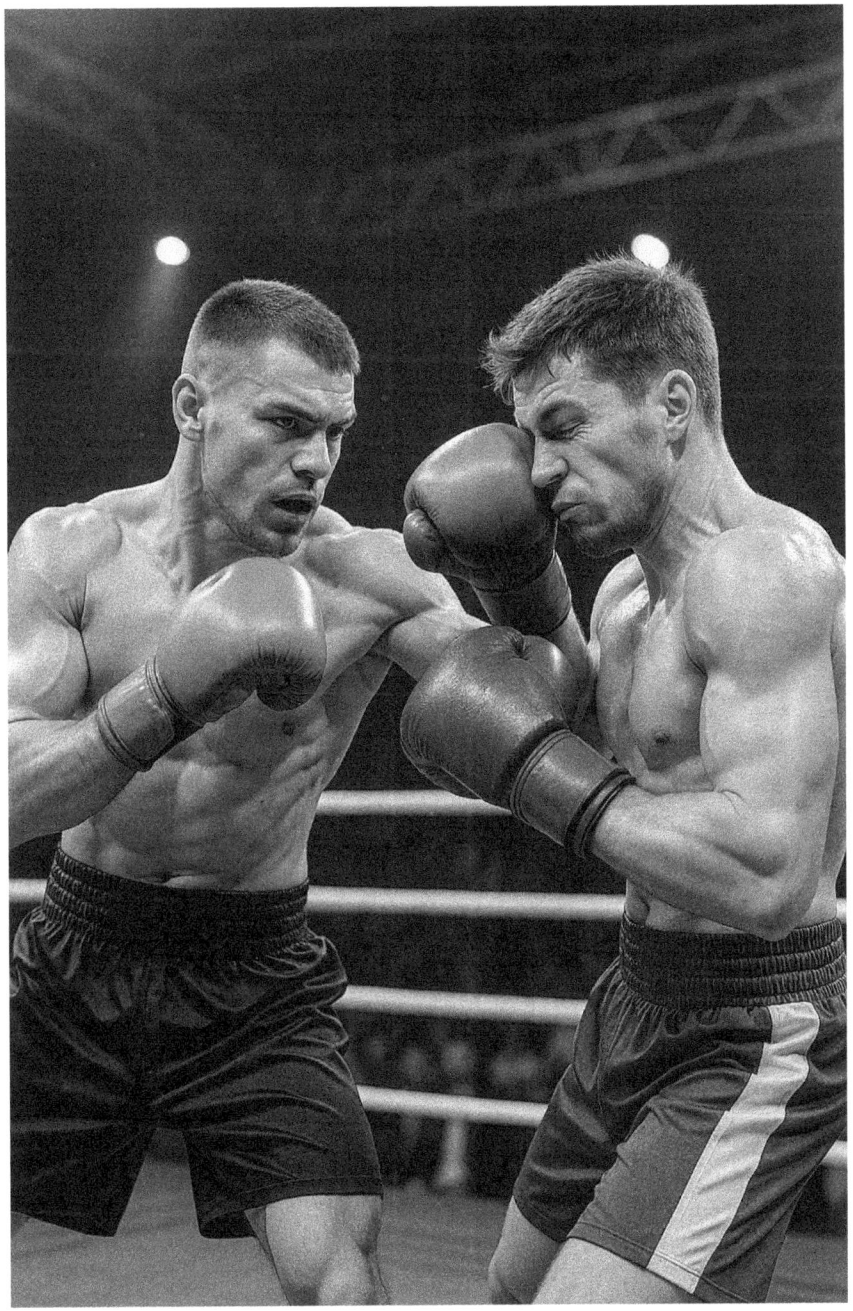

3. Combat Sports (Boxing, MMA)

Combat sports like **boxing** and **MMA** are some of the most intense and physically demanding forms of training. They build unmatched conditioning, mental toughness, and practical self-defense skills. But because of their intensity and full-contact nature, they also come with risks and require responsible training. Understanding both the benefits and drawbacks helps athletes train safely and effectively.

◈ Benefits (PLUS)

1. Exceptional Full-Body Conditioning
Boxing and MMA engage almost every major muscle group:

- Legs (movement, kicks, footwork)
- Core (punch power, stability, grappling)
- Upper body (punching, clinching, submissions)

These sports improve strength, agility, balance, and flexibility all at once.

2. Incredible Cardiovascular Fitness
Combat sports elevate the heart rate rapidly.
Rounds of striking, grappling, and movement create high-intensity interval training (HIIT), improving:

- Heart health
- Lung capacity
- Endurance
- Overall stamina

Few sports match the conditioning level of combat training.

3. Practical Self-Defense Skills

Boxing teaches striking, footwork, distancing, and timing. MMA combines:

- Boxing
- Kickboxing
- Wrestling
- Jiu-jitsu
- Grappling

These skills provide effective real-world self-defense ability and personal confidence.

4. Builds Mental Toughness & Discipline

Combat sports demand:

- Focus
- Confidence
- Controlled aggression
- Patience
- Strategic thinking

Athletes learn emotional control, resilience, and the ability to stay calm under pressure — valuable traits in life.

5. Major Stress Relief

Punching, kicking, or grappling is a powerful outlet for:

- Stress
- Frustration
- Anxiety

Endorphins released during training boost mood and reduce tension.

6. Strong Community & Respect Culture
Combat gyms emphasize respect, humility, and discipline. Training partners often form strong friendships and team spirit.

◈ Drawbacks (MINUS)

1. Risk of Injury
Because of full contact, common injuries include:

- Bruises and cuts
- Sprains and strains
- Shoulder or wrist injuries
- Concussions (especially in heavy sparring)
- Joint injuries from grappling

Safe training and good coaching greatly reduce risks.

2. High Physical Demands
Combat sports require intense conditioning. Beginners may find:

- Workouts extremely tiring
- Muscle soreness frequent
- Recovery time longer

Athletes must balance hard training with proper rest.

3. Requires Skilled Coaching

Poor technique increases injury risk dramatically. Proper instruction is essential for:

- Punching form
- Kicking mechanics
- Grappling safety
- Defensive skills

Good gyms can also be more expensive.

4. Potential for Overtraining

Fighters often push themselves too hard, leading to:

- Fatigue
- Burnout
- Weakened immune system
- Loss of motivation

Structured training plans prevent this.

5. Not Always Beginner-Friendly

MMA and boxing can be intimidating for new athletes due to:

- Contact
- Fast pace
- Complex techniques
- Intensity of sparring

However, beginner classes exist in most gyms.

6. Long-Term Wear and Tear

Heavy sparring over many years may increase:

- Joint stress
- Chronic pain
- Risk of head injuries

Moderate sparring and good technique help protect long-term health.

Summary

Combat sports like boxing and MMA provide some of the best full-body training available. They improve strength, endurance, agility, confidence, and real self-defense ability. But their intensity requires good coaching, proper technique, and responsible training habits to avoid injury and burnout.

When practiced safely, combat sports are one of the most powerful ways to develop both physical and mental strength.

4. Flexibility & Mobility Sports (Yoga, Gymnastics)

Flexibility and mobility sports like **yoga** and **gymnastics** focus on controlled movement, balance, stretching, and body awareness. These activities improve the body's ability to move freely, prevent injuries, and build long-lasting strength and stability. While these sports offer many physical and mental benefits, they also require proper technique and progression to avoid strain or injury.

◈ Benefits (PLUS)

1. Increases Flexibility and Range of Motion

Yoga and gymnastics stretch muscles, tendons, and ligaments, allowing joints to move more freely.
Improved flexibility helps:

- Reduce stiffness
- Improve posture
- Prevent injuries
- Enhance physical performance in all other sports

2. Builds Strong, Lean Muscles

Many yoga poses and gymnastics movements rely on bodyweight resistance.
This strengthens:

- Core
- Shoulders
- Back
- Legs
- Stabilizing muscles

These sports develop long, balanced, and functional strength rather than bulky muscle.

3. Improves Balance, Coordination & Body Control

Gymnastics teaches precise movement, while yoga enhances balance and stability.
This improves:

- Motor control
- Agility
- Awareness of body position

- Joint stability

These skills prevent falls and enhance athletic performance.

4. Enhances Mental Focus and Stress Relief

Yoga especially promotes:

- Mindfulness
- Deep breathing
- Relaxation
- Mental clarity

Both sports require concentration, which helps reduce anxiety, improve mood, and increase emotional stability.

5. Supports Injury Prevention and Recovery

Flexible muscles and mobile joints reduce the risk of strain or tears. Yoga is often used in rehabilitation programs to:

- Improve circulation
- Release muscle tension
- Restore mobility after injury

6. Excellent for Posture and Spinal Health

Stretching tight muscles in the neck, shoulders, and back corrects posture.
This reduces:

- Back pain
- Tension headaches
- Muscle imbalances

◈ Drawbacks (MINUS)

1. Risk of Overstretching or Joint Strain
Too much flexibility without proper strength can lead to:

- Ligament overstretching
- Joint instability
- Hip or shoulder pain

Beginners often push too hard, causing strain.

2. Requires Patience and Long-Term Consistency
Flexibility improvements take time.
Some people may feel discouraged if progress is slow, especially in gymnastics where skills can take months or years.

3. Not Always Beginner-Friendly (Especially Gymnastics)
Gymnastics includes advanced movements such as:

- Handstands
- Cartwheels
- Rings
- Flips

These require coaching and gradual progression to avoid injury.

4. Potential for Wrist, Shoulder, or Back Stress
Frequent weight-bearing on hands (common in gymnastics and yoga) may cause:

- Wrist soreness
- Shoulder strain
- Lower back pressure

Proper technique and strengthening are essential.

5. Flexibility Without Strength Can Create Imbalance
Some individuals stretch more than they strengthen.
This can lead to:

- Weak stabilizer muscles
- Poor joint support
- Increased injury risk

Balance between stretching and strength is crucial.

6. Requires Good Instruction
Incorrect form can lead to injuries, especially in deep poses or advanced gymnastics.
Good coaching or guided classes help avoid poor habits.

Summary

Flexibility and mobility sports like yoga and gymnastics offer powerful benefits: improved flexibility, strong core and stabilizer muscles, better posture, enhanced balance, and mental calmness. However, like all sports, they require proper technique, gradual progression, and a balanced approach to prevent overstretching or joint strain.

When practiced safely and consistently, these sports greatly improve overall athletic ability, mobility, and long-term physical health.

4

Building a Fitness Routine

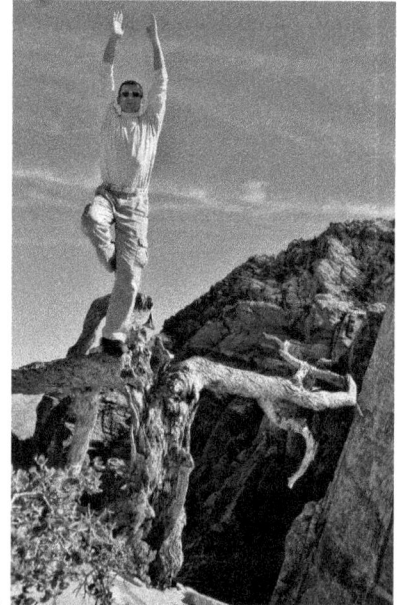

1.

Warm-Up & Stretching

Warm-up and stretching are essential parts of any safe and effective fitness routine. They prepare the body for physical activity, reduce the risk of injury, improve performance, and support long-term mobility and joint health. Many people skip these steps, but they are just as important as the workout itself. A proper warm-up and stretching routine ensures that the body moves smoothly, safely, and efficiently.

A **warm-up** gradually increases heart rate, blood flow, and body temperature. When your muscles warm up, they become more flexible and responsive, allowing them to contract and relax more efficiently. This prepares the cardiovascular system for the demands of exercise and ensures that the joints move with better lubrication and stability. A good warm-up also activates the nervous system, improving coordination, balance, and reaction time — all critical for sports that require fast movements and agility.

Stretching, especially dynamic stretching before exercise, helps lengthen muscles and improve range of motion. When muscles are tight or stiff, they limit your mobility and increase the chance of strains, pulls, and joint stress. Stretching reduces muscle tension, improves posture, and enhances the efficiency of movement. It prepares the body to perform more naturally and reduces the likelihood of sudden injuries during training or sports.

During warm-ups, the body slowly shifts from a resting state to an active state. The lungs begin to deliver more oxygen, the heart starts pumping more efficiently, and the brain becomes more alert. This transition helps athletes feel more prepared mentally as well, reducing anxiety and increasing focus. Proper warm--ups improve the quality of the workout and allow athletes to move at full power without shock to the muscles or joints.

After exercise, **static stretching** is important for recovery. It helps cool the body down, reduces muscle soreness, and improves flexibility over time. Stretching after workouts releases built-up tension, promotes circulation, and allows the body to return to a relaxed state. Maintaining flexibility supports better posture and prevents long-term stiffness that can build up from repetitive training.

Skipping warm-ups and stretching can lead to injuries such as muscle strains, ligament sprains, joint irritation, or decreased performance. Cold muscles are more prone to tearing, and sudden movements without preparation place unnecessary stress on the body.

In summary, warm-up and stretching are essential components of healthy, safe, and effective training. They improve performance, protect the body from injury, prepare the mind for activity, and support long-term mobility and recovery. Making these steps a consistent part of your routine ensures that you build strength, flexibility, and endurance in a safe and balanced way.

2. Training Frequency & Volume

Training frequency and training volume are two of the most critical factors that determine progress, performance, and long-term health in any fitness routine. **Frequency** refers to how often you train each week, while **volume** refers to how much total work you perform — sets, repetitions, distance, duration, or intensity. Balancing these two elements ensures that the body adapts correctly, grows stronger, and stays healthy without breaking down from overtraining or inactivity.

Training frequency is important because the body requires **consistent stimulation** to improve. Whether the goal is strength, endurance, flexibility, or general fitness, muscles and cardiovascular systems respond best to repeated, regular activity. Training only once in a while is not enough to create lasting changes. Regular movement improves circulation, regulates metabolism, strengthens muscles, and helps maintain a healthy body weight. Consistency is what transforms exercise into a lifestyle rather than a temporary habit.

Training volume determines the **total stress** placed on the body. Too little volume leads to slow progress, while too much volume can cause fatigue, injury, and burnout. The right amount of volume challenges the muscles and cardiovascular system enough to trigger adaptation, but not so much that it overwhelms the body. A balanced volume improves strength, increases stamina, and enhances athletic performance without overloading joints, tendons, or the nervous system.

Both frequency and volume also play a major role in **recovery**. When these factors are properly balanced, the body has enough time to repair muscle tissue, replenish energy stores, and strengthen bones and connective tissues. Without this balance, the risk of overtraining increases — leading to exhaustion, sleep problems, decreased performance, and a weakened immune system. Properly planned training schedules help avoid these issues and allow steady, long-term progress.

In terms of health, training frequency and volume support long-term **heart health, metabolic function, and mobility**. Regular activity helps regulate blood pressure, control blood sugar, improve cholesterol levels, and strengthen the heart. Adequate volume ensures the body receives enough challenge to stay strong and flexible, which supports healthy aging and reduces the risk of chronic diseases.

Psychologically, consistent training frequency builds **motivation, discipline, and mental clarity**. Meanwhile, the right volume prevents burnout and keeps exercise enjoyable rather than exhausting. This balance helps people stay committed to fitness goals for years, not just weeks.

In summary, training frequency and training volume are essential because they control how the body adapts, how fast you progress, and how safely you train. When balanced correctly, they improve physical strength, cardiovascular health, metabolism, and overall well-being. The right combination of frequency and volume creates a sustainable routine that keeps the body strong, energized, and healthy for life.

3. How to Choose the Right Sport

Choosing the right sport is one of the most important decisions for building a healthy, enjoyable, and long-lasting fitness routine. The ideal sport matches your interests, physical ability, personality, goals, and lifestyle. When you choose a sport that fits you, staying consistent becomes natural — and consistency is the key to lifelong health. The right sport not only improves your body but also strengthens your mind, boosts motivation, and supports emotional well-being.

The first step in choosing the right sport is understanding your **fitness goals**. If you want to build strength and muscle, sports like weightlifting, wrestling, or rowing may be ideal. If your goal is endurance, running, cycling, or swimming are excellent choices. For full-body conditioning and skill development, team sports like soccer or basketball are effective. If flexibility and stress relief are priorities, yoga or martial arts may be the right fit. Your goals guide you toward activities that support your physical needs.

Next, consider your **personality and interests**. Some people enjoy the excitement, teamwork, and social interaction of team sports, while others prefer the focus and independence of solo activities. If you love competition, fast-paced sports may motivate you. If you prefer calm, controlled movement, yoga, Pilates, or recreational swimming may be more satisfying. Enjoyment is one of the strongest predictors of long-term success — if you enjoy the activity, you will return to it again and again.

Your **physical abilities and limitations** also matter. Individuals with joint issues may benefit from low-impact sports such as cycling, swimming, or walking. Those with strong coordination might excel in ball sports, while people with natural strength may enjoy power-based sports. Choosing a sport that suits your current physical condition prevents injuries and builds confidence as you progress.

Another important factor is **accessibility** — time, equipment, facilities, and cost. Running requires only shoes and open space. Weightlifting needs a gym or basic equipment. Team sports require fields, courts, or scheduled practices. Choosing a sport that fits your lifestyle increases consistency and decreases excuses.

It is also helpful to think about **progression and learning style**. Some sports are simple to start, such as jogging, cycling, or walking. Others require technique and coaching, such as martial arts, gymnastics, or tennis. Selecting a sport that matches your desire to learn new skills ensures long-term engagement and satisfaction.

Finally, it's important to **listen to your body and experiment**. Try different sports until you find the one that feels right. A sport that energizes you, challenges you, and leaves you excited for the next session is the perfect match. The right sport makes training enjoyable, sustainable, and deeply rewarding.

In summary, choosing the right sport involves understanding your goals, interests, abilities, lifestyle, and personality. When you select a sport that fits who you are, you build a routine that strengthens the body, sharpens the mind, and improves your overall quality of life.

4. **Structuring Your Weekly Plan.**

Structuring your weekly plan is essential for creating a balanced, effective, and sustainable approach to fitness. Without a clear plan, workouts can become inconsistent, unbalanced, or even risky. A weekly plan gives your body the right combination of activity, rest, and progression — all of which are necessary for achieving long-term health. When your exercise routine is properly organized, you improve faster, feel better, and protect your body from avoidable setbacks.

A structured weekly plan ensures **balanced training**, which means you train all major parts of fitness — strength, endurance, flexibility, and recovery. Many people focus only on one area, such as cardio or weightlifting, and neglect the others. This imbalance can lead to plateaus, posture issues, joint stress, or reduced performance. A well-planned week includes different types of workouts, giving your body everything it needs to function at its best.

Planning your week also helps manage **training load**, which includes both frequency and volume. Too much exercise without proper rest can cause fatigue, injury, and burnout. Too little exercise slows progress and weakens motivation. When you organize your weekly schedule, you can place intense workouts on certain days and lighter sessions or rest on others. This allows your muscles and nervous system to recover, grow stronger, and adapt safely.

Another major benefit is improved **consistency**. Having a plan removes guesswork and helps you avoid skipping workouts. You know exactly what you need to do each day, which builds discipline and turns exercise into a habit instead of a chore. Consistency is the number one factor that determines long-term health success — even more than workout intensity.

A weekly plan also supports **smarter progression**. Progress happens gradually, not all at once. A structured schedule lets you track your workouts, increase difficulty safely, and measure improvements over time. This prevents stagnation and keeps training motivating and enjoyable. It also helps you adjust your plan based on your goals, whether you want to lose weight, gain muscle, improve endurance, or increase mobility.

Finally, structuring your week benefits **mental and emotional health**. Planning reduces stress and helps you feel organized and in control. You can include workouts you enjoy, schedule recovery time, and avoid last-minute decisions that lead to inconsistency. Knowing your plan gives your mind clarity and your body stability.

In summary, structuring your weekly plan is important because it ensures balanced training, prevents injury, builds consistency, encourages steady progress, and supports both physical and mental well-being. A well-planned week creates a strong foundation for lifelong health and fitness success.

5

Strength Training for Everyone

1. Muscle Growth Basics

Muscle growth, also known as **hypertrophy**, is the process by which the body increases the size, strength, and endurance of muscle fibers. This happens when the muscles experience stress through resistance training, repair themselves, and adapt to become stronger than before. Understanding the basics of muscle growth helps you train more effectively, avoid injury, and build long-lasting strength.

Muscle growth begins when you challenge your muscles with **resistance or weight**, such as lifting dumbbells, using machines, doing bodyweight exercises, or performing challenging sports. When the muscle fibers work harder than they are used to, tiny microscopic tears form in the tissue. These tears are not harmful — they are the signal the body needs to start the rebuilding process. During recovery, the body repairs these fibers, making them thicker, denser, and stronger. This is how strength and muscle size increase over time.

To stimulate growth, muscles need **progressive overload** — gradually increasing the weight, intensity, or number of repetitions. Without progression, the body will stop improving because it adapts quickly. Even small increases, such as adding a few pounds, doing one more repetition, or slowing down the movement, help keep the muscles challenged and growing.

Another key element of muscle growth is **proper form and full range of motion**. Good technique ensures that the correct muscles are activated and protected from injury. When exercises are performed with control and full extension, more muscle fibers are engaged, improving growth and functional strength.

Nutrition plays an essential role in making muscles stronger. Muscles require **protein** to repair damaged fibers. Eating protein-rich foods such as chicken, fish, eggs, beans, and dairy supports recovery and growth. Carbohydrates provide energy for workouts, while healthy fats support hormone balance — especially hormones like testosterone and growth hormone, which are crucial for muscle development.

Rest and recovery are just as important as training. Muscles do not grow during the workout — they grow afterward, when the body is repairing them. Without proper rest, the body cannot fully recover, which limits progress and increases fatigue. Getting enough sleep, spacing out training days, and allowing muscle groups time to heal all help maximize strength gains.

Consistency is the foundation of muscle development. Strength increases gradually over weeks and months, not overnight. When you train regularly, fuel your body properly, and allow it to recover, you will continuously build muscle and get stronger.

In summary, muscle growth is driven by challenging the muscles with resistance, using progressive overload, maintaining good technique, eating proper nutrients, and allowing enough recovery time. When these key principles work together, the body becomes stronger, more powerful, and more capable — supporting long-term health, performance, and confidence.

2. Core Strength

Core strength is one of the most important foundations of overall health, fitness, and movement. The core is not just the "abs" — it includes the muscles of the stomach, lower back, hips, obliques, and deep stabilizers around the spine. These muscles work together to support posture, protect the spine, stabilize the body, and allow nearly every movement you make. A strong core improves performance in sports, daily activities, and even simple tasks such as walking, lifting, and bending.

The core is the **center of the body's strength and stability**. Every movement — whether pushing, pulling, jumping, or twisting — begins with the core. When the core is weak, other muscles must compensate, which increases the risk of injury. A strong core keeps the spine aligned, improves posture, reduces lower-back pain, and helps the body maintain balance when moving or standing. Core strength is especially crucial for preventing injuries during physical activity, as it stabilizes joints and protects the spine during sudden movements.

Core strength also improves **athletic performance**. In sports like running, soccer, basketball, wrestling, boxing, and gymnastics, the core transfers power from the lower body to the upper body. A strong core increases speed, agility, balance, and explosive power. Even in non-athletic activities, such as carrying groceries, climbing stairs, or getting out of bed, the core is constantly working to stabilize the body.

A strong core also supports **breathing and digestion**, as core muscles assist the diaphragm during deep breathing and help maintain proper internal pressure. This contributes to better endurance, healthier organs, and improved circulation.

Developing core strength does not require heavy equipment. Many effective exercises use only body weight. Some of the most beneficial core exercises include:

1. Planks

Strengthens the deep core muscles, lower back, glutes, and shoulders.
Hold for 20–60 seconds with proper form.

2. Leg Raises

Targets the lower abs and hip flexors. Perform slowly for maximum control.

3. Russian Twists

Strengthens the obliques and improves rotational stability.

4. Bird-Dog

Excellent for spine alignment and lower-back protection.

5. Mountain Climbers

Builds core endurance and improves cardio fitness.

6. Dead Bug

Strengthens the deep stabilizer muscles and teaches proper coordination.

7. Glute Bridge

Strengthens the glutes and lower back, both crucial parts of the core.

Consistency is key. Training the core two to four times a week is enough to build strength without overworking the muscles. Proper form is essential, as rushing through exercises can strain the lower back. Slow, controlled movements activate the core more effectively than fast repetitions.

In summary, core strength is important because it stabilizes the body, protects the spine, improves posture, enhances athletic performance, and prevents injuries. With consistent practice and simple exercises, anyone can build a strong, stable, and healthy core that supports the entire body's movement and wellbeing.

3. Training with Weights

Training with weights is one of the most effective ways to build strength, improve overall fitness, and support long-term health. Weight training challenges the muscles in ways that everyday movement cannot. It creates resistance that forces the body to grow stronger, denser, and more resilient. Whether using dumbbells, barbells, kettle bells, or machines, weight training is a powerful tool for improving physical performance and protecting the body as it ages. However, because it involves added resistance and stress on muscles and joints, proper technique and caution are essential for safe, long-term progress.

Weight training is important because it **builds muscle mass**, which plays a major role in strength, mobility, and metabolism. Strong muscles help support joints, stabilize the body, and make daily activities easier — from lifting groceries to climbing stairs. As people age, they naturally lose muscle, a process called sarcopenia. Weight training slows and even reverses this loss, keeping the body functional and independent. More muscle also increases metabolism, helping burn more calories even at rest, which aids in weight control and fat loss.

Another major benefit of weight training is **improved bone density**. When you lift weights, the stress placed on bones stimulates them to grow stronger and denser. This reduces the risk of osteoporosis, fractures, and bone weakness later in life. Weight training also enhances posture, balance, and joint stability by strengthening the muscles around the spine, hips, knees, and shoulders.

Weight training boosts **athletic performance** as well. Increased strength improves speed, power, endurance, and agility in nearly every sport. Even for people who are not athletes, weight training improves confidence, energy levels, and long-term resilience.

However, because weight training involves higher levels of resistance, it must be done carefully. The most important safety rule is **proper form**. Lifting too heavy or using incorrect technique increases the risk of injuries such as muscle strains, joint irritation, herniated discs, or tendon problems. Beginners should start with light to moderate weights and learn the correct movement patterns before increasing intensity.

Another safety factor is **progressive overload** — gradually increasing weight, sets, or repetitions. Jumping too quickly to heavy loads can overwhelm the body. Slow, consistent progression builds strength safely and effectively. It is also essential to **warm up** before lifting and **rest between sets** to maintain good form and avoid fatigue-related injuries.

Listening to your body is equally important. Sharp pain, joint discomfort, or unusual strain are signals to stop and reassess your technique or weight selection. Recovery — including adequate sleep, hydration, and rest days — is crucial, because muscles grow stronger after training, not during it.

In summary, training with weights is important because it builds muscle, strengthens bones, boosts metabolism, improves posture, supports joint health, and enhances athletic ability. With proper technique, gradual progression, and smart safety habits, weight training becomes one of the most powerful and beneficial forms of exercise for lifelong health and strength.

4. Bodyweight-Only Strength Training

Bodyweight-only strength training is a highly effective and accessible way to build muscle, improve fitness, and strengthen the entire body — all without needing weights or gym equipment. By using your own body as resistance, you can increase strength, balance, mobility, and endurance anywhere, anytime. This training method is ideal for beginners, travelers, home workouts, or anyone who wants safe, functional strength development.

Bodyweight exercises work by challenging your muscles through **movement patterns** such as pushing, pulling, squatting, lifting, and stabilizing. When performed correctly, they activate the same muscle groups used in weight training, helping build lean muscle and improve overall athletic performance. Because the resistance is your own body, the joints experience less stress than with heavy weights, making this style of training safer and easier to start.

The foundation of bodyweight training includes exercises such as:

1. Push-Ups

Strengthen the chest, shoulders, triceps, and core.
Variations include incline, decline, wide-arm, or diamond push-ups to adjust difficulty.

2. Squats

Target the quadriceps, glutes, hamstrings, and core.
Advanced versions include jump squats, single-leg squats, or wall sits for increased challenge.

3. Lunges

Improve leg strength, balance, and stability.
Reverse, walking, and lateral lunges provide variety.

4. Planks

Build core strength, posture, and shoulder stability.
Side planks and extended planks increase intensity.

5. Pull-Ups or Inverted Rows

If a pull-up bar is available, these build the back and biceps.
Without equipment, you can use doorframe bars or table rows.

6. Dips

Strengthen chest, shoulders, and triceps using parallel bars, chairs, or benches.

7. Glute Bridges

Activate the glutes and lower back, important for posture and hip stability.

To get the most benefit from bodyweight strength training, you should follow key principles:

• Progressive Overload

Even without weights, you must gradually increase difficulty. This can be done by:

- Adding more repetitions
- Increasing time under tension
- Trying harder variations
- Slowing down the movement
- Reducing rest time between sets

• Full Range of Motion

Move your joints through their complete movement path. This develops strength evenly and improves mobility.

• Control and Technique

Slow, controlled movements activate muscles more effectively and prevent injury.
Proper form matters more than speed or repetition count.

• Balanced Training

Include pushing, pulling, leg, and core movements to prevent muscle imbalances.

A simple and effective bodyweight workout might include:

- 3 sets of push-ups
- 3 sets of squats
- 3 sets of lunges
- 1–2 minutes of planks
- 3 sets of glute bridges
- Light stretching afterward

Bodyweight training is highly adaptable. You can make it easier for beginners or extremely challenging for advanced athletes by modifying angles, tempo, and positioning.

In summary, bodyweight-only strength training is a powerful, convenient, and safe way to build muscle and improve fitness. With consistency, progression, and proper technique, anyone can achieve strong, functional, and balanced muscles using nothing more than their own body.

6

Cardio for Health & Fat Loss

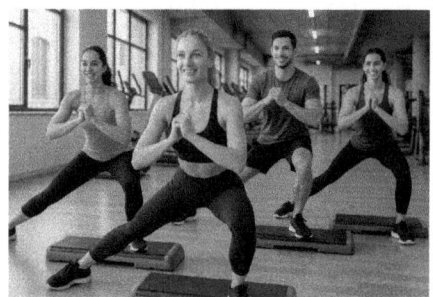

1. Low-Intensity Cardio

Low-intensity cardio is one of the most effective and sustainable forms of exercise for improving health, burning fat, and increasing overall endurance. It involves performing activities at a comfortable, steady pace where your heart rate increases but you can still breathe and talk easily. This type of cardio is safe for all ages and fitness levels, making it perfect for beginners, seniors, and those recovering from injury. Low-intensity cardio strengthens the heart and lungs without putting excessive stress on the joints or nervous system.

Low-intensity cardio is performed at **50–65% of your maximum heart rate**. A simple guideline is the **"talk test"**: if you can talk comfortably during the activity, you are in the correct zone. The key is maintaining a steady pace for an extended period, usually **20–60 minutes**. This helps improve circulation, increases oxygen use, and trains the body to burn fat efficiently.

Here are some of the best examples of low-intensity cardio:

1. Walking
Walking is the most accessible and beginner-friendly form of low-intensity cardio.
Benefits include improved heart health, better mobility, and reduced stress.
Aim for a brisk but comfortable pace.

2. Light Jogging or Slow Running
For those who enjoy running, a slow, relaxed pace qualifies as low intensity.
This builds stamina without overwhelming the joints or muscles.

3. Cycling at an Easy Pace
Outdoor biking or stationary cycling at low resistance is excellent for joint-friendly cardio.
It strengthens the legs and improves cardiovascular endurance.

4. Swimming or Water Walking
Water provides natural resistance while supporting the body, making it perfect for people with joint issues.
Gentle swimming laps or walking in shallow water count as low-intensity work.

5. Elliptical Trainer
Using an elliptical machine at low resistance and moderate speed offers a smooth, low-impact workout for the entire body.

6. Hiking on Flat Trails
Hiking on flat or slightly inclined paths combines walking with the benefits of fresh air and nature.
This improves mood, endurance, and heart health.

7. Rowing at a Light Pace

Rowing machines provide full-body cardio with minimal impact. Keep resistance low and focus on steady rhythm.

8. Dance or Aerobic Movement

Light dance sessions, low-impact aerobics, and rhythmic movement routines are enjoyable ways to keep your heart rate up without stress.

To get results from low-intensity cardio, consistency is key. Aim for **3–5 sessions per week**, gradually increasing the duration as your fitness improves. This type of training is ideal for burning fat, improving metabolism, reducing stress, and improving overall cardiovascular health. Because it is gentle on the body, it can be performed more frequently than high-intensity workouts.

Low-intensity cardio also pairs well with strength training. It helps warm up the body, promotes recovery, and improves endurance without interfering with muscle growth.

In summary, low-intensity cardio is an accessible, safe, and effective way to improve heart health, increase stamina, and support weight management. Through simple activities like walking, cycling, swimming, or light jogging, anyone can achieve significant health benefits while maintaining a comfortable, enjoyable workout routine.

2. High-Intensity Interval Training (HIIT)

High-Intensity Interval Training, commonly known as **HIIT**, is one of the most time-efficient and powerful forms of exercise for improving fitness, burning fat, and boosting heart health. HIIT alternates short bursts of intense effort with brief periods of rest or low-intensity movement. This style of training pushes the body to work harder than steady-pace cardio, creating fast improvements in endurance, strength, and metabolism. Because HIIT is adaptable to any fitness level, it can be done at home, in the gym, or outdoors.

HIIT works by raising your heart rate quickly during intense intervals, then allowing it to drop during recovery periods. A simple structure is **20–40 seconds of high effort followed by 20–40 seconds of rest**, repeated for several rounds. The intensity during the work phase should feel challenging — fast breathing, elevated heart rate — but still safe and controlled. HIIT sessions are typically **10–25 minutes** long, making them ideal for busy people who want maximum results in minimum time.

Here are some effective HIIT exercises you can combine:

1. Sprints
Run fast for 20–30 seconds, walk or jog for 30–60 seconds. Boosts leg power and cardiovascular strength.

2. Jumping Jacks
A full-body movement that increases heart rate quickly. Perfect for beginners.

3. Burpees
A powerful exercise combining squats, planks, and jumps. Excellent for strength and cardio together.

4. High Knees
Drive knees upward rapidly for a fast cardio burst.

5. Mountain Climbers
Engage the core and shoulders while raising heart rate.

6. Cycling Sprints
Pedal hard for 15–30 seconds, then slow down for recovery. A basic HIIT workout might look like this:

- 30 seconds: high-intensity exercise (sprint, burpees, etc.)

- 30 seconds: rest or slow movement
- Repeat for 10–15 minutes

HIIT can be done with bodyweight, machines, dumbbells, or simple movements — as long as intensity goes up during each work period.

◈ Benefits of HIIT

1. Burns More Calories in Less Time

HIIT is extremely efficient. Short sessions burn as many calories as long traditional workouts, making it ideal for fat loss and busy schedules.

2. Boosts Metabolism After the Workout

HIIT triggers the "afterburn effect" (EPOC), causing the body to burn extra calories for hours after training.
This helps with weight control and fat reduction.

3. Improves Cardiovascular and Lung Health

Short, intense bursts strengthen the heart and improve oxygen use. Over time, HIIT increases endurance and overall fitness dramatically.

4. Builds Strength and Muscle Endurance

Many HIIT exercises engage multiple muscle groups at once.
This improves functional strength, coordination, and power.

5. Requires No Equipment

HIIT can be performed anywhere — at home, in a park, or in the gym.
Simple movements like squats and sprints make it accessible for all levels.

6. Increases Mental Toughness

Pushing through short intense intervals builds discipline, focus, and confidence.

7. Time-Efficient and Versatile

Workouts can be as short as 10 minutes but still highly effective. Great for people with limited time.

Summary

HIIT is a fast, powerful, and efficient training method that improves strength, endurance, heart health, and fat loss. It requires no equipment, fits into any schedule, and can be adjusted for beginners or advanced athletes. With proper form, controlled intensity, and consistent effort, HIIT provides some of the most impressive health and fitness benefits of any exercise style.

3. Improving Lung Capacity

Improving lung capacity is essential for better breathing, higher endurance, stronger athletic performance, and overall health. The lungs play a major role in supplying oxygen to the body and removing carbon dioxide. When lung capacity increases, your body delivers oxygen more efficiently, allowing you to move longer, breathe easier, and feel more energized during daily activities. Whether you are an athlete, someone starting fitness, or a person wanting to breathe better, lung training is one of the most valuable health investments you can make.

Lung capacity improves when you challenge your respiratory system with controlled breathing exercises, cardiovascular activity, and posture training. The goal is to strengthen the diaphragm, expand the lungs more fully, and increase oxygen flow throughout the body. Just like muscles, lungs respond to consistent training and grow more efficient over time.

How to Improve Lung Capacity

1. Diaphragmatic (Belly) Breathing

This exercise strengthens the diaphragm and encourages deeper, fuller breaths.

How to do it:

- Lie down or sit upright.
- Place one hand on your chest and one on your stomach.
- Inhale slowly through the nose, pushing your belly outward.
- Exhale through the mouth, letting your belly fall.
  Repeat for 5–10 minutes daily.

2. Pursed-Lip Breathing

Helps control airflow and improves oxygen exchange.

How to do it:

- Inhale deeply through your nose for 2–3 seconds.
- Exhale slowly through pursed lips (like blowing out a candle) for 4–6 seconds.
  This strengthens the lungs and calms the breathing system.

3. Breath-Holding Exercises

These help increase lung volume and oxygen capacity.

How to do it:

- Inhale deeply for 4 seconds.
- Hold for 4–8 seconds.
- Exhale slowly.
  Repeat 5–10 cycles.

4. Aerobic Exercise

Consistent cardio improves lung strength and endurance.
Examples:

- Walking
- Jogging
- Cycling
- Swimming
- Rowing

Aim for **20–45 minutes**, 3–5 times a week.

Effective Lung-Building Activities

1. Running or Jogging

Improves oxygen use, strengthens breathing muscles, and increases overall capacity.

2. Swimming

Water resistance forces deeper breathing and strengthens the diaphragm.
One of the most powerful ways to build lung function.

3. HIIT Cardio

Short bursts of intense work increase oxygen demand, training the lungs to respond quickly.

4. Singing or Wind Instruments

Activities like singing, playing flute, trumpet, or harmonica expand lung control and breath volume.

5. Yoga & Deep Breathing Poses

Yoga focuses on long inhalation and exhalation, improving lung flexibility, relaxation, and airflow.

6. Stair Climbing

Strengthens legs while forcing deeper breathing, improving both endurance and lung capacity.

Why Lung Capacity Matters

Better lung capacity improves:

- Athletic performance
- Heart health
- Energy and stamina
- Recovery after exercise
- Ability to manage stress
- Breathing efficiency
- Overall quality of life

Stronger lungs mean more oxygen for your muscles, brain, and organs — allowing you to live more actively and comfortably.

Summary

Improving lung capacity requires consistent practice of breathwork, aerobic exercise, and posture control. Through simple techniques like diaphragmatic breathing, cardio training, and yoga, anyone can expand their lung strength and boost endurance. The result is better breathing, improved performance, and long-lasting health benefits.

4. Heart Health Benefits

A healthy heart is essential for a long, energetic, and active life. The heart is the engine of the body, pumping oxygen-rich blood to every organ, muscle, and tissue. When the heart functions efficiently, the entire body performs better — from physical endurance and strength to mental clarity and emotional well-being. Achieving strong heart health requires a combination of exercise, proper nutrition, smart lifestyle choices, and daily habits that keep the cardiovascular system strong.

Why Heart Health Matters

A healthy heart improves **circulation**, delivering oxygen and nutrients more efficiently. This results in higher energy levels, faster recovery, and better stamina during everyday activities and workouts. A strong heart also reduces the risk of serious conditions such as high blood pressure, stroke, heart attacks, and artery disease. Heart health is one of the biggest factors affecting longevity — people with healthier cardiovascular systems live longer, more active lives.

Good heart function also supports **mental health**. Healthy blood flow improves brain oxygenation, helping you think clearly, stay focused, and maintain emotional balance. Better circulation also improves sleep quality, mood, and overall stress resistance.

What You Need to Do for Heart Health Benefits

Improving heart health involves consistent physical activity, mindful eating, and healthy daily habits. Here are the most effective steps:

1. Do Regular Cardio Exercise

Cardiovascular activity trains the heart to pump blood more efficiently.
Effective cardio includes:

- Walking
- Jogging
- Cycling
- Swimming
- Dancing
- Rowing

Aim for **150 minutes of moderate** or **75 minutes of vigorous cardio per week.**

2. Add High-Intensity Interval Training (HIIT)

HIIT improves heart strength and oxygen use more quickly than traditional cardio.

Short bursts of intense effort followed by rest help:

- Lower blood pressure
- Improve circulation
- Increase heart efficiency

3. Strength Training

Lifting weights or doing bodyweight exercises supports the heart by reducing fat, increasing muscle, and improving metabolism.

Perform strength training **2–3 times a week.**

4. Eat Heart-Healthy Foods

Nutrition plays a major role in cardiovascular health. Focus on:

- Vegetables and fruits
- Whole grains
- Lean proteins
- Healthy fats (olive oil, nuts, avocados)
- Omega-3 rich foods (fish, flaxseed)

Reduce foods that stress the heart:

- Excess salt

- Fried or processed foods
- Sugary snacks
- Excess alcohol

5. Maintain a Healthy Weight

Less body fat reduces strain on the heart.
Combining exercise with balanced nutrition helps maintain a healthy weight naturally.

6. Manage Stress

Chronic stress increases blood pressure and heart strain.
Use techniques such as:

- Deep breathing
- Meditation
- Yoga
- Walking in nature
- Good sleep habits

7. Avoid Smoking

Smoking damages blood vessels and decreases oxygen delivery.
Quitting immediately improves heart health and circulation.

Summary

Heart health benefits are achieved through consistent cardio exercise, smart nutrition, strength training, stress management, and healthy lifestyle habits. Improving your heart function enhances energy, stamina, brain health, emotional stability, and overall longevity. By making heart-focused choices daily, you protect your most important organ — creating a stronger, healthier, and more vibrant life.

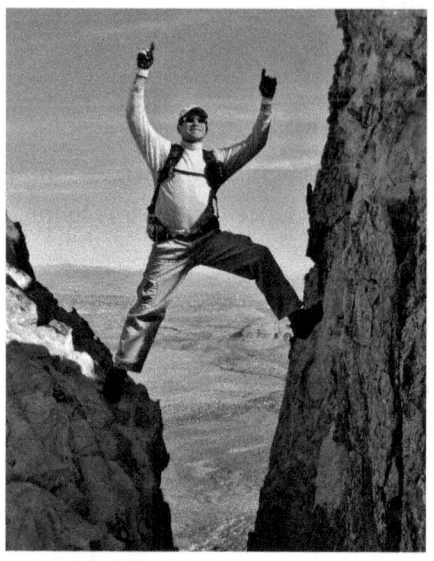

Why Hiking in Mountains & Parks Helps With Depression, Weight Loss, and Health

Hiking is one of the most powerful natural therapies for both the body and mind. Walking through mountains, forests, and national parks combines physical exercise with the healing effects of nature. This combination reduces stress, burns calories, improves mood, strengthens the heart, and restores mental clarity. Hiking is more than a workout — it is a full-body and full-mind experience that improves overall well-being.

1. Hiking Helps Fight Depression

Nature has a scientifically proven positive effect on mental health. When you hike:

- **Stress drops immediately**

Trees, fresh air, sunlight, and natural quiet lower cortisol — the body's stress hormone.
This creates calmness and mental relief.

- **Your brain chemistry improves**

Hiking boosts endorphins and serotonin, the "feel-good" chemicals that help fight anxiety and depression.

- **Negative thoughts slow down**

Walking in peaceful environments reduces overthinking and mental noise.
Nature acts like a natural reset button for the mind.

- **You feel connected, not isolated**

Mountains and parks make people feel grounded and part of something bigger, reducing feelings of loneliness.

- **Sunlight boosts mood**

Sunlight increases vitamin D and regulates sleep cycles, both important for mood stability.

2. Hiking Helps With Weight Loss

Hiking is one of the most effective and enjoyable ways to burn calories without feeling like hard exercise.

- **Burns more calories than regular walking**

Steep hills, uneven ground, and long trails activate more muscles — especially legs, core, and glutes.

- **Increases metabolism**

The body works harder on uneven terrain, boosting calorie burn during and after the hike.

- **Easy to stay consistent**

Unlike gym workouts, hiking is fun and scenic.
When exercise feels enjoyable, people do it more often — which leads to real weight loss.

- **Builds lean muscle**

Climbing hills strengthens muscles, which increases metabolism and helps burn fat faster.

3. Benefits of Walking in Nature

Walking in nature benefits the entire body, mind, and spirit.

Physical Benefits
- Improves heart and lung health
- Reduces blood pressure
- Strengthens joints and muscles
- Increases energy levels
- Supports healthy aging

Mental Benefits
- Enhances creativity and focus
- Reduces anxiety
- Improves sleep
- Clears the mind
- Boosts overall happiness

Emotional & Spiritual Benefits
- Creates peace and a sense of calm
- Deepens connection to the world
- Encourages gratitude and mindfulness
- Helps release emotional tension

4. Why Hiking Is So Effective

Hiking is powerful because it combines **exercise + nature + mindfulness** all at once:

- Exercise heals the body
- Nature heals the mind
- Mindfulness heals the emotions

This triple combination makes hiking one of the most complete and natural forms of therapy.

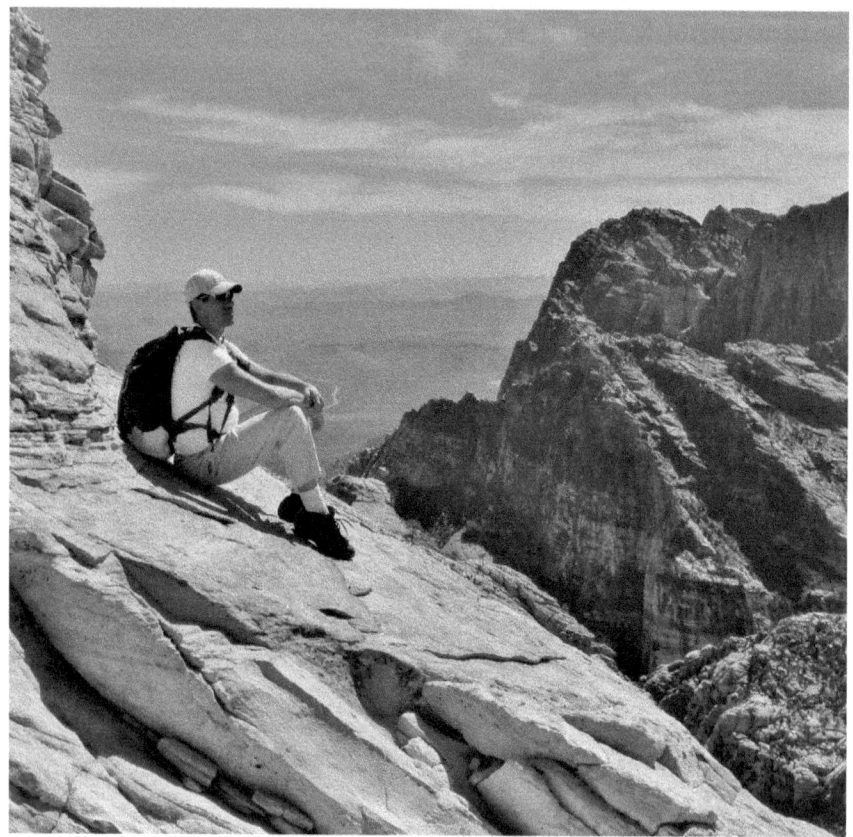

Summary

Hiking in mountains and parks helps with depression by reducing stress, improving mood, and calming the mind. It supports weight loss through natural calorie burning, increased metabolism, and enjoyable movement. Walking in nature improves physical health, emotional well-being, and mental clarity. Hiking is not just an outdoor activity — it is a holistic path to a healthier, happier, and stronger life.

7

Nutrition for Sports Performance

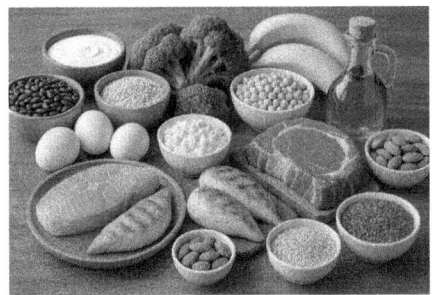

1. Proteins, Carbs & Fats

Proper nutrition is the foundation of health, energy, and physical performance. Every food you eat contains macronutrients — **protein**, **carbohydrates**, and **fats** — which provide the fuel your body needs to move, repair, and function. Each macronutrient plays a different role, and all three are essential. Understanding why they matter and how to choose healthy sources helps you build strength, maintain energy, and support long-term well-being.

1. Protein – The Body's Building Material

Why Protein Is Important

Protein is essential for building and repairing tissues throughout the body.
It supports:

- Muscle growth
- Recovery after exercise
- Strong bones
- Healthy skin, hair, and nails
- Immune system function
- Hormone production

For athletes or active people, protein is crucial for rebuilding muscle fibers after workouts.

Examples of Healthy Proteins

- Chicken, turkey
- Fish (salmon, tuna, sardines)
- Eggs
- Greek yogurt
- Cottage cheese
- Beans and lentils
- Tofu and tempeh
- Nuts and seeds

Aim for protein at every meal to support muscle repair and energy balance.

2. Carbohydrates – The Body's Main Energy Source

Why Carbs Are Important

Carbohydrates are the body's preferred source of energy. They fuel:

- Workouts and sports performance
- Brain function and concentration
- Muscle power
- Daily activities (walking, working, thinking)

Carbs also help maintain steady blood sugar levels, preventing fatigue and mood crashes.

Inadequate carbs can lead to low energy, poor performance, and difficulty building muscle.

Examples of Healthy Carbs

- Oats
- Brown rice
- Whole wheat bread
- Potatoes and sweet potatoes
- Fruits (bananas, apples, berries)
- Vegetables
- Quinoa
- Beans

Choose complex carbs that digest slowly and provide lasting energy.

3. Fats – Essential Fuel and Hormone Support

Why Healthy Fats Are Important

Fats are often misunderstood, but they are essential for:

- Hormone balance (testosterone, estrogen, growth hormones)
- Brain function and mood
- Joint lubrication
- Vitamin absorption (A, D, E, K)
- Long-lasting energy

Healthy fats help keep you full, protect organs, and stabilize blood sugar.

Examples of Healthy Fats
- Avocados
- Olive oil
- Nuts (almonds, walnuts)
- Seeds (chia, flax, pumpkin)
- Fatty fish (salmon, mackerel)
- Coconut oil (used moderately)
- Natural peanut or almond butter

Avoid unhealthy fats such as trans fats found in fried and processed foods.

Summary

Protein builds and repairs the body, carbohydrates fuel it, and healthy fats support hormones, energy, and brain function. Each macronutrient is essential — removing one creates imbalance, fatigue, or health problems. Eating a balanced mix of proteins, carbs, and fats provides sustained energy, supports muscle strength, and promotes long-term health and performance.

2. Hydration

Hydration is one of the most important, yet often overlooked, factors in maintaining good health, physical performance, and mental function. Water makes up about 60% of the human body and is involved in nearly every biological process. Without proper hydration, the body cannot function at its best — even small drops in water levels can affect energy, mood, strength, and brain performance. Staying hydrated is essential for longevity, athletic ability, and everyday well-being.

Water is crucial for **regulating body temperature**. When you move, exercise, or spend time in warm environments, your body produces heat. Sweat cools the body and prevents overheating — but sweating also removes water and minerals. Without proper hydration, your body struggles to cool down, leading to fatigue, dizziness, and increased risk of heat exhaustion. Drinking enough water keeps your internal temperature balanced and safe.

Hydration is also vital for **muscle function and physical performance**. Muscles contain a high percentage of water, and dehydration can cause cramps, weakness, and slower reaction times. Even mild dehydration reduces strength, endurance, and coordination. Athletes and active individuals especially rely on hydration to keep muscles energized and maintain peak performance.

The **brain** depends heavily on water. Proper hydration improves focus, memory, mood, and mental clarity. Dehydration, even at low levels, can cause headaches, irritability, poor concentration, and slower thinking. Staying hydrated nourishes the brain and supports healthy nerve function.

Water is essential for **digestion and nutrient absorption**. It helps break down food, transport nutrients through the bloodstream, and support kidney function. When the body lacks water, digestion slows, leading to constipation, bloating, and reduced nutrient absorption. Adequate hydration keeps the digestive system smooth and efficient.

Hydration plays a major role in **energy levels**. Many people feel tired not because of lack of sleep or food, but because they are dehydrated. Water helps the body convert food into energy and ensures oxygen reaches cells. Without enough water, energy production decreases, resulting in fatigue and sluggishness.

Proper hydration also supports **healthy skin, joint lubrication,** and **detoxification.** Water helps remove waste from the body through urine and sweat. It keeps joints cushioned, reducing the risk of pain and stiffness. Hydrated skin appears smoother, healthier, and more elastic.

To stay properly hydrated, aim to drink water consistently throughout the day. Most people benefit from **6–10 cups daily**, with more needed during exercise, hot weather, or illness. Sports drinks or electrolytes may help replace minerals lost through heavy sweating, but plain water is the most important factor.

In summary, hydration is vital because it regulates temperature, fuels muscles, supports the brain, improves digestion, boosts energy, protects joints, and removes toxins. Drinking enough water every day is one of the simplest and most powerful habits for a healthier, stronger, and more energized life.

3. Pre-Workout Nutrition

Pre-Workout Nutrition: Importance and Examples

Pre-workout nutrition is essential for fueling your body before exercise, boosting performance, and protecting your muscles from fatigue and breakdown. What you eat before training directly affects your strength, endurance, energy levels, and mental focus. Without proper pre-workout fuel, the body struggles to perform at its best, leading to early exhaustion, weaker workouts, and slower progress over time.

The main goal of pre-workout nutrition is to provide **energy, hydration,** and **nutrients** that support your muscles during exercise. Carbohydrates give you quick and reliable fuel by raising blood sugar and delivering energy to the muscles. Protein supports muscle repair and prepares your body for recovery. Healthy fats can also be helpful for longer, low-intensity sessions, but are less essential for fast, intense workouts.

Eating the right food before exercise improves **performance** by increasing stamina, strength, and focus. When your body has fuel, you can push harder, lift heavier, and stay mentally sharp throughout your training session. Pre-workout nutrition also helps prevent dizziness, nausea, and muscle breakdown caused by training on an empty stomach. For people aiming for muscle growth, eating before a workout provides amino acids that protect your muscle fibers during intense physical stress.

Timing is important. Ideally, eat a balanced snack or small meal **30–90 minutes before exercise**. Eating too close to your workout can cause stomach discomfort, while eating too early may leave you without enough energy. The perfect timing varies by person, but the goal is to feel light, energized, and ready to move.

Examples of Good Pre-Workout Foods

Carbohydrate + Protein Combinations

These provide quick energy and muscle support.

- Banana with peanut butter
- Greek yogurt with berries
- Oatmeal with honey
- Whole-grain toast with turkey or egg
- Rice cakes with almond butter
- Fruit smoothie with protein powder

Light, Fast-Digesting Options

Great for workouts starting soon.

- Banana or apple

- Small granola bar
- Handful of dried fruit
- Coconut water for quick hydration

More Complete Pre-Workout Meals (60–90 minutes before)

Suitable before longer or intense sessions.

- Chicken with rice
- Eggs with whole-grain toast
- Tuna and crackers
- Cottage cheese with fruit

Hydration Before Training

Drink water **15–30 minutes before** starting.
For long or intense workouts, add electrolytes for better hydration and muscle function.

Summary

Pre-workout nutrition is important because it boosts energy, improves performance, prevents fatigue, supports muscle strength, and prepares the body for recovery. Eating the right combination of carbohydrates, protein, and hydration ensures that your workouts are stronger, safer, and more effective. With proper pre-workout fuel, you train harder, feel better, and make greater progress toward your fitness goals.

If you want, I can continue with:

4. Post-Workout Recovery

Post-workout recovery is a crucial part of any fitness routine. After exercise — whether strength training, cardio, or sports — the body needs time to repair muscle fibers, restore energy, and reduce physical stress. Recovery is not optional; it is when the actual progress happens. Without proper recovery, muscles cannot grow, the body cannot adapt, and performance gradually decreases. Prioritizing recovery is essential for long-term health, strength, and injury prevention.

During exercise, especially intense training, tiny tears form in the muscle fibers, and energy stores such as glycogen are depleted. Recovery allows the body to repair these tears, rebuild muscle stronger than before, and replenish lost nutrients. The cardiovascular system also needs time to return to normal levels, and the nervous system must recover from stress. When recovery is skipped or rushed, the body becomes fatigued, increasing the risk of injury, soreness, and burnout.

Post-workout recovery is also important for reducing inflammation and preventing chronic fatigue. Proper rest helps regulate hormones like cortisol, improves sleep quality, and supports immune function. Athletes who recover well experience better strength gains, improved endurance, and more consistent performance across training sessions.

How Long Does Recovery Take?

Recovery time depends on the type and intensity of the workout:

1. Light Exercise (walking, stretching, easy cardio)
Recovery time: A few hours

Light activities require minimal recovery. The body can return to normal quickly.

2. Moderate Cardio or Strength Training
Recovery time: 24–48 hours
Most general workouts need one to two days for muscles to repair and energy to refill.

3. Intense Strength Training (heavy lifting, HIIT, explosive sports)
Recovery time: 48–72 hours
Muscles worked intensely need more time for healing and rebuilding.

4. Very Intense or High-Volume Training (long runs, intense sports, leg day)
Recovery time: 72 hours or more
Large muscle groups, especially legs, may need extra time before training them again.

Recovery is not only about waiting — the following practices speed up and improve the process:

Key Components of Effective Recovery

1. Nutrition
Eat a combination of protein and carbohydrates within **30–90 minutes** after exercise.
Examples: chicken and rice, protein shake with fruit, yogurt with granola.

2. Hydration
Replace water and electrolytes lost during sweating to help muscles function properly.

3. Sleep

Quality sleep (7–9 hours) is the most powerful recovery tool. The body repairs tissue and releases growth hormones while you sleep.

4. Stretching and Mobility

Light stretching reduces tension, improves flexibility, and speeds muscle repair.

5. Rest Days

Planned rest days allow muscles and the nervous system to reset.

6. Active Recovery

Gentle movement such as walking, easy cycling, or yoga increases blood flow and reduces soreness.

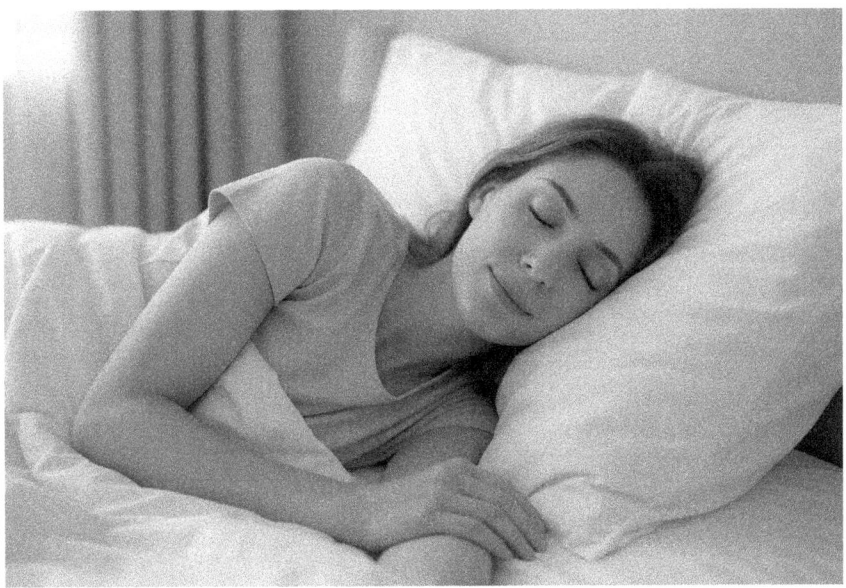

Summary

Post-workout recovery is important because it repairs muscles, restores energy, reduces inflammation, and prevents injury. Most workouts require **24–72 hours** of recovery depending on intensity. With proper nutrition, sleep, hydration, and rest, your body becomes stronger after every training session, leading to faster progress and better long-term health.

8

Mental Benefits of Sports

Sports also improve **blood flow to the brain**, delivering more oxygen and nutrients that help enhance memory, concentration, and mental clarity. Regular physical activity stimulates the growth of new brain cells in areas connected to learning and emotional regulation. This makes your mind sharper, more focused, and more resilient.

Participating in sports builds **self-confidence** and a positive self-image. When you reach fitness goals, learn new skills, or improve performance, you feel a sense of accomplishment. This boosts self-esteem and teaches you that you are capable of growth and improvement. Sports also help you develop discipline, accountability, and mental toughness — qualities that carry into school, work, and daily life.

Sports are also powerful for **stress relief**. Physical activity acts as a healthy outlet for frustration, worry, or emotional tension. Whether it's lifting weights, running, swimming, or playing team sports, movement helps clear your mind and release negative emotions. After exercise, people often feel more relaxed, patient, and mentally refreshed.

Team sports add another layer of mental benefit: **social connection**. Being part of a team provides a sense of belonging, trust, communication, and support. These positive social relationships improve emotional stability and reduce feelings of loneliness or isolation. Even solo sports foster social interaction through classes, gyms, or training groups.

Regular sports participation also improves **sleep quality**, which is essential for mental health. Better sleep helps regulate mood, improves creativity, and enhances decision-making. People who exercise regularly fall asleep faster, sleep deeper, and wake up more refreshed.

Finally, sports help build **emotional resilience**. Challenging workouts teach you how to push through discomfort, stay calm under pressure, and overcome setbacks. This mental strength translates into everyday life, helping you handle stress, face difficulties, and maintain a positive outlook.

Summary

Sports support mental health by releasing feel-good chemicals, reducing stress, sharpening focus, improving confidence, and building emotional resilience. Physical activity strengthens the body and the mind, creating a healthier, calmer, and more motivated you — making sports one of the most powerful tools for lifelong mental well-being.

1. Stress & Anxiety Relief

Sports and fitness activities are among the most effective natural tools for reducing stress and managing anxiety. When you move your body, powerful physical, chemical, and emotional changes take place that calm the mind, release tension, and restore balance. Regular physical activity reshapes how the brain responds to daily pressure and helps you become stronger mentally as well as physically.

One of the main ways fitness reduces stress is through the release of **endorphins**, often called the "feel-good hormones." These natural chemicals act as the body's own antidepressants, lifting your mood and creating a sense of positivity and relaxation. Exercise also lowers the levels of **cortisol**, the primary hormone released during stress. When cortisol stays high for too long, it can lead to anxiety, irritability, and fatigue.

By reducing cortisol, exercise helps the mind return to a calmer, more grounded state.

Sports and fitness also improve **breathing patterns**, which directly influence emotional well-being. Activities like running, cycling, swimming, or even brisk walking increase oxygen flow and encourage deeper, more rhythmic breathing. This stimulates the parasympathetic nervous system — the part of the body responsible for calm and relaxation. With improved breathing, your heart rate lowers, your body tension decreases, and your mind becomes clearer.

Physical activity provides an important **mental break** from everyday worries. When you are focused on your movements, breathing, or the rhythm of your workout, your attention shifts away from negative thoughts. This mental distraction helps interrupt cycles of over thinking and anxiety. Many athletes notice that training becomes a form of meditation where they process emotions and leave stress behind.

Sports also build **confidence and emotional resilience**. Each time you complete a workout, learn a new skill, or push through a challenging exercise, your brain receives a message: *I can overcome difficulty.* This mindset strengthens your ability to handle pressure in daily life. Over time, your stress response becomes less reactive and more controlled.

Another major benefit comes from **social interaction**. Team sports, group fitness classes, and workout partners create a sense of connection and support. Positive social experiences naturally reduce stress levels and help prevent feelings of loneliness — a major contributor to anxiety.

Regular exercise improves **sleep quality**, which is essential for emotional stability. Better sleep helps regulate mood, increases patience, and improves your ability to cope with stressful situations. People who exercise consistently fall asleep faster, sleep deeper, and wake up more refreshed, reducing anxiety throughout the day.

Finally, physical activity teaches **healthy coping strategies**. Instead of turning to unhealthy habits like overeating, isolation, or avoidance, exercise becomes a proactive outlet for releasing frustration and calming the mind.

Summary

Sports and fitness reduce stress and anxiety by releasing feel-good chemicals, lowering cortisol, improving breathing, providing mental clarity, boosting confidence, and improving sleep. Whether it's running, lifting, yoga, or team sports, regular physical activity strengthens your emotional resilience and helps you stay calm, balanced, and mentally strong.

2. Confidence Building

Sports and fitness are powerful tools for developing self-confidence. Confidence does not appear overnight — it grows through action, consistency, and personal achievement. Physical activity strengthens the body, but it also shapes the mind, teaching discipline, resilience, and self-belief. The challenges and victories experienced in sports help build a strong internal foundation of confidence that carries into all areas of life.

One of the biggest ways sports build confidence is by creating **visible progress**. When you train consistently, you become stronger, faster, and more skilled. You notice changes in your endurance, body shape, strength, and overall ability. These improvements show you that your hard work is paying off. This sense of progress proves that you can achieve goals through effort — a powerful confidence booster.

Sports and fitness also help you overcome **self-doubt**. Every time you finish a workout, complete a difficult set, or learn a new movement, you demonstrate to yourself that you are capable of more than you thought. This builds mental resilience and teaches you to trust your own abilities. You learn that you can push through challenges, which increases belief in yourself both during exercise and in everyday situations.

Regular physical activity improves **posture, energy, and body image**, all of which strongly influence confidence. Standing taller, feeling stronger, moving easier, and having more energy naturally make you feel better about yourself. Exercise also releases endorphins, improving mood and helping you feel more positive and motivated. A healthier body often leads to a healthier self-image, reducing insecurity and boosting self-esteem.

Sports give you opportunities to set **goals and achieve them**. Whether it's lifting a heavier weight, running a faster mile, improving flexibility, or mastering a technique, each achievement reinforces your confidence. Goal-setting in fitness teaches you how to measure progress, celebrate small wins, and stay motivated even when challenges arise.

Team sports add another layer to confidence building through **social interaction**. Working with teammates, receiving support, and contributing to group success increases your sense of belonging and social confidence. Even in solo sports, training communities and fitness classes create encouragement, accountability, and positive reinforcement.

Sports also teach **discipline and mental toughness**. Confidence grows when you prove to yourself that you can stay committed, show up consistently, and maintain focus under pressure. These skills translate directly into work, school, relationships, and other areas of life, making you more assertive and self-assured.

Finally, fitness provides a powerful sense of **control and empowerment**. When you invest in your health, overcome obstacles, and build physical strength, you feel more capable in all aspects of life. This sense of empowerment boosts self-worth and helps you approach challenges with confidence rather than fear.

Summary

Sports and fitness build confidence by creating progress, strengthening mental resilience, improving body image, teaching discipline, and providing social support. Through consistent effort and achievement, athletes learn to trust themselves, overcome challenges, and develop a strong, positive sense of who they are.

3. Discipline & Motivation

Sports and fitness are some of the most powerful tools for developing discipline and motivation. These qualities are not fixed traits — they grow when you practice consistency, face challenges, and commit to personal improvement. Training the body naturally trains the mind, and the habits built through regular exercise become the foundation for a more focused, responsible, and motivated life.

One of the biggest ways sports build discipline is through **routine**. When you commit to exercising regularly — whether it's three times a week or every day — you teach yourself to follow a schedule, even when you don't feel like it. Showing up repeatedly builds mental strength. Over time, the body adapts, the mind adapts, and discipline becomes easier and more automatic.

Sports also help develop discipline by teaching **responsibility and self-control**. Strength training, running, martial arts, and team sports require proper technique, good choices, and respect for your own physical limits. To improve, you must follow training plans, rest when needed, eat properly, and stay consistent. These habits strengthen self-control and teach you how to make decisions that support your goals rather than short-term comfort.

Fitness also builds motivation through **visible progress**. When you start seeing results — stronger muscles, better stamina, more flexibility, improved speed, or weight loss — it fuels your desire to keep going. Progress, even small progress, motivates you to push harder. Each improvement proves that your effort matters, creating a positive cycle: **the more you do, the more you want to do**.

Sports develop **mental toughness**, another form of discipline. Hard workouts teach you how to push through discomfort, deal with setbacks, and keep going when challenges arise. Learning to push past your limits in training helps you become more resilient in everyday life — whether facing work stress, personal challenges, or long-term goals.

Motivation also grows through **goal setting**. Whether it's lifting heavier weights, running faster, achieving a personal record, or learning a new skill, sports help you set short-term and long-term goals. Working toward these goals teaches planning, focus, and persistence. Achieving goals increases confidence and creates momentum, making you even more motivated to continue.

Team sports add an additional motivational boost through **community and accountability**. Teammates, coaches, or training partners create support and encouragement. When others rely on you, you naturally become more disciplined. Even in solo fitness, classes, gyms, and online communities help keep motivation high.

Sports and fitness also improve motivation by **reducing stress, improving mood, and increasing energy**. When you feel better mentally and physically, it becomes easier to stay motivated in all areas of life. Regular exercise boosts endorphins and improves sleep, both of which help you stay focused and driven.

Summary

Sports and fitness build discipline and motivation through routine, responsibility, progress, goal-setting, mental toughness, and social support. Training strengthens both the body and the mind, helping you become more focused, consistent, and driven — not just in exercise, but in every part of your life.

4. Social and Emotional Health

Sports and fitness activities are powerful tools not only for physical development, but also for strengthening social connections and emotional well-being. Whether through team sports, group fitness classes, or even individual exercise done in shared environments, physical activity provides numerous benefits that support healthier relationships, improved emotional balance, and a greater sense of belonging. These mental and social benefits make sports an effective long-term strategy for overall life satisfaction and emotional resilience.

One of the biggest impacts of sports on social health comes from **community and connection**. When you join a sports team, fitness class, running group, or gym community, you meet people with similar goals and interests. These connections reduce loneliness, increase feelings of belonging, and create supportive relationships. Humans are social by nature, and participating in shared physical activities builds trust, cooperation, and communication skills.

Sports also improve emotional health by creating **positive interactions** and meaningful social experiences. Celebrating victories, encouraging teammates, and learning to work together all build emotional strength. In group settings, people often feel supported, valued, and motivated. These social bonds help reduce stress and improve mood, making fitness a powerful emotional outlet.

Physical activity also boosts emotional stability through **chemical changes** in the brain. Exercise releases endorphins — natural mood enhancers — and reduces cortisol, the stress hormone. This leads to a calmer mind, fewer negative thoughts, and better emotional balance. Many people experience improved patience, confidence, and happiness after regular exercise.

Sports provide a healthy way to express emotions. Physical activity allows you to release frustration, anxiety, or sadness in a safe and productive manner. Workouts serve as emotional "reset buttons," helping clear your mind and process feelings more effectively. Over time, this helps you develop healthier emotional coping strategies.

Another major benefit is improved **self-esteem and self-image**. Achieving fitness goals, learning new skills, and seeing physical progress help you feel more confident about yourself. Confidence leads to better communication, stronger social connections, and a more positive emotional outlook.

Team sports also teach valuable **social skills** such as cooperation, leadership, listening, and empathy. Working with teammates builds understanding and emotional intelligence. These skills transfer into relationships, careers, and daily life, helping you interact more effectively with others.

Sports and fitness also improve **emotional resilience**. Training regularly teaches you how to handle setbacks, stay calm under pressure, and bounce back from challenges. This resilience strengthens both emotional and social health, helping you maintain better relationships and make healthier decisions.

Finally, fitness promotes **better sleep**, **higher energy**, and **reduced anxiety**, all of which support emotional stability and positive social interactions. When you feel good mentally and physically, you communicate better, engage more, and connect more deeply with others.

Summary

Sports and fitness improve social and emotional health by creating community, boosting confidence, reducing stress, enhancing emotional resilience, and developing important relationship skills. Through movement and shared experiences, physical activity strengthens both the mind and the heart — helping you feel happier, more connected, and more emotionally balanced.

9

Injury Prevention & Healing

1. How to Warm Up Properly

A proper warm-up prepares your body for exercise by increasing blood flow, raising muscle temperature, activating joints, and improving movement quality. Warming up reduces the risk of injury, improves performance, and mentally prepares you for the workout ahead. A good warm-up should take **5–10 minutes** and gradually transition your body from rest to activity.

A complete warm-up has **three key parts**: (1) gentle movement, (2) dynamic stretching, and (3) sport-specific activation.

1. Start With Light Movement (2–3 minutes)

This step increases heart rate and warms the muscles.

Examples:
- Brisk walking
- Easy jogging
- Light cycling
- Jumping jacks
- Marching in place
- Slow rowing

This improves blood flow and prepares your joints for more intense motion.

2. Dynamic Stretching (2-3 minutes)

Dynamic stretches activate muscles through controlled movement — not holding a position.
They improve flexibility, range of motion, and coordination.

Examples:
- **Leg swings** (front/back and side-to-side)
- **Arm circles** (small to large)
- **Hip circles**
- **Torso twists**
- **Walking lunges**
- **High knees**
- **Butt kicks**

Dynamic stretching wakes up muscles and increases joint mobility in preparation for activity.

3. Sport-Specific Activation (2-4 minutes)

This step prepares the exact muscles you will use during your workout.
You mimic your upcoming movements but with lower intensity.

Examples Based on Workout Type:
For Strength Training:
- Light squats
- Push-up walkouts

- Glute bridges
- Resistance-band rows
- Shoulder activation with bands

For Running:
- Light jog + stride-outs
- A-skips or B-skips
- Calf raises
- Short acceleration runs

For Sports (basketball, soccer, etc.):
- Dribbling or ball control
- Short sprints
- Agility steps
- Side shuffles

For HIIT:
- Slow burpees
- Easy mountain climbers
- Slow step-outs
- Joint mobility drills

Activation improves coordination, muscle firing, and reaction time.

Putting It All Together (Sample 5-Minute Warm-Up)

Minute 1–2:
Light jog or brisk walk
Minute 3–4:
Dynamic stretches:

- Arm circles
- Leg swings
- Hip rotations
- Walking lunges

Minute 5:

Sport-specific activation:

- 10 bodyweight squats
- 10 push-ups
- 20 jumping jacks

This simple routine effectively prepares the entire body.

Summary

A proper warm-up increases blood flow, improves mobility, protects your joints, and boosts performance. By combining light movement, dynamic stretching, and sport-specific activation, your body becomes ready for safe, strong, and effective exercise. A good warm-up makes every workout better.

2. Common Injuries & How to Avoid Them

Sports and fitness activities offer enormous physical and mental benefits, but without proper technique, preparation, and recovery, injuries can occur. Understanding the most common injuries and how to prevent them is essential for staying healthy, consistent, and confident in your fitness routine. Most injuries are avoidable with smart training habits — and learning how to protect your body ensures long-term success and safety.

Common Sports & Fitness Injuries

1. Muscle Strains
What they are: Overstretching or tearing of muscle fibers, commonly in the hamstrings, quadriceps, shoulders, or back.
Causes: Poor warm-up, sudden movements, lifting too heavy, or lack of flexibility.

2. Sprains
What they are: Overstretching or tearing of ligaments, usually in the ankles, wrists, or knees.
Causes: Quick direction changes, jumping, unstable surfaces.

3. Tendonitis
What it is: Inflammation of a tendon caused by repetitive stress.
Common areas: Elbows, knees, shoulders, Achilles tendon.
Causes: Overuse, poor technique, and lack of rest.

4. Knee Pain (Runner's Knee / Patellar Issues)
What it is: Pain around the kneecap from overuse or poor leg alignment.
Causes: Weak hips, overtraining, improper footwear.

5. Back Pain
What it is: Strain or irritation of spinal muscles or discs.
Causes: Lifting with poor form, weak core, sudden twisting.

6. Shin Splints
What they are: Pain along the shinbone from repetitive impact.
Causes: Running too much too soon, hard surfaces, poor shoes.

7. Shoulder Injuries

Common injuries: Rotator cuff strain, impingement.
Causes: Overhead lifting, poor posture, weak stabilizers.

How to Avoid These Injuries

1. Warm Up Properly

A good warm-up increases blood flow, activates muscles, and prepares joints.
Always include:

- Light cardio
- Dynamic stretching
- Sport-specific activation

2. Use Proper Technique

Poor form is one of the biggest causes of injury.
Learn correct movement patterns, especially for:

- Lifting weights
- Running
- Jumping
- Rotational movements

If unsure, start light or ask a coach for guidance.

3. Progress Gradually

Avoid "too much, too soon."
Increase:

- Weight
- Speed

- Distance
- Duration
  Slowly and progressively.

4. Strengthen Supporting Muscles

Injury-prone areas often suffer from weak stabilizers. Focus on:

- Core strength
- Hip stability
- Shoulder rotator cuff
- Glute muscles
- Strong supporting muscles protect joints.

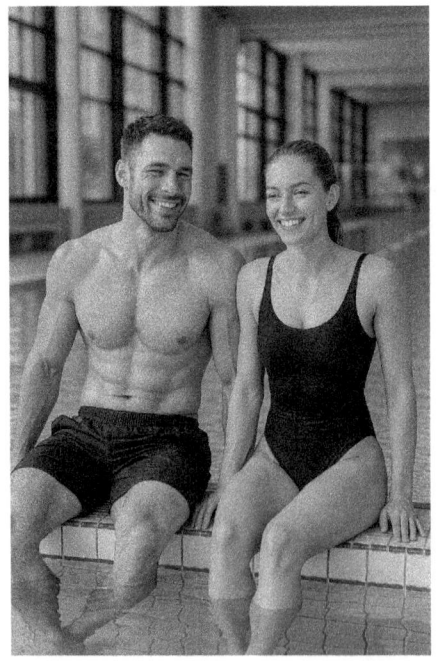

5. Rest and Recover

Muscles repair during rest, not during workouts.
Take rest days and prioritize:

- Sleep
- Hydration
- Light stretching
- Active recovery

Overtraining leads to injury.

6. Use Proper Equipment

The right shoes, supportive gear, and well-maintained equipment reduce impact stress and improve safety.
Replace worn-out shoes regularly.

7. Listen to Your Body

Sharp pain, swelling, or unusual discomfort is a warning sign.
Stop immediately, rest, and adjust your training plan.

Summary

Most sports and fitness injuries — including sprains, strains, tendonitis, knee pain, and back issues — result from poor technique, overtraining, or lack of preparation. By warming up properly, using good form, progressing gradually, strengthening stabilizers, and prioritizing recovery, you can avoid injuries and train safely for life. Injury prevention is not just about staying safe — it's about building a stronger, more resilient body.

When to Rest

Rest is one of the most important parts of health, fitness, and overall well-being. Many people focus only on training, but **rest is when your body actually heals, grows, and becomes stronger**. Without proper rest, performance drops, injuries increase, and mental and physical stress begin to build. Understanding when and why your body needs rest is essential for long-term success in both sports and daily life.

Your body needs rest **whenever it has been placed under stress** — through exercise, work, or emotional demands. During physical activity, muscles experience tiny tears, energy levels drop, and the nervous system becomes fatigued. Rest allows the body to repair these tissues, restore energy, and rebalance hormones. Without rest, the body cannot rebuild itself, leading to exhaustion and weaker performance.

Rest is especially important after **intense workouts**, such as strength training, HIIT, long runs, heavy sports activity, or any movement that pushes your muscles and cardiovascular system. These workouts require **24–72 hours** for full repair depending on intensity. Training too soon without recovery increases the risk of injury, soreness, and burnout.

Your body also needs rest when you feel **unusually tired**, mentally drained, or unable to focus. Physical fatigue and mental fatigue are connected. If sleep quality drops or stress levels rise, your performance during workouts and daily tasks declines. Rest helps restore mental clarity, emotional balance, and motivation.

Sleep is the most powerful form of rest. During **7–9 hours of quality sleep**, your body releases growth hormones, repairs tissues, strengthens the immune system, and resets the nervous system. Without enough sleep, reaction time, strength, endurance, and mood all suffer. Your metabolism slows, cravings increase, and your risk of illness or injury grows.

There are different types of rest your body needs:

1. Physical Rest

Time off from intense exercise to allow muscle repair and joint recovery.
Examples: rest days, lighter workouts, stretching.

2. Mental Rest

Breaks from stress, work, or overstimulation.
Examples: quiet time, nature walks, meditation.

3. Sleep-Based Rest

Deep restorative sleep that rebuilds the body and mind.

4. Active Recovery

Light movement that increases blood flow without stressing the body.
Examples: walking, gentle yoga, light cycling.

Your body also signals when it needs rest:

- Persistent soreness
- Low energy
- Mood changes
- Trouble sleeping
- Slow recovery
- Decreased performance
- Increased heart rate even at rest

Listening to these signals prevents long-term damage.

Summary

Your body needs rest because it repairs muscles, restores energy, balances hormones, strengthens the immune system, and protects your physical and mental health. Proper rest — including sleep, rest days, and mental downtime — ensures you stay strong, motivated, injury-free, and able to perform at your best. Rest is not the opposite of training — **it is an essential part of training**.

3. Healing Through Movement

Healing through movement is a powerful method of restoring physical, mental, and emotional well-being. Instead of complete rest or inactivity, the body often recovers faster when it performs gentle, controlled, and purposeful movement. This concept — known as **active recovery** — improves circulation, reduces stiffness, relaxes the mind, and encourages the body to repair itself naturally. Movement is medicine, and when used correctly, it can accelerate healing and improve long-term mobility, strength, and confidence.

How Healing Through Movement Works

When you move lightly, your body increases **blood flow** to muscles, joints, and tissues. This delivers oxygen and nutrients needed for repair, while removing waste products that cause soreness and stiffness. Gentle movement also helps reduce inflammation, improve joint lubrication, and restore normal range of motion. For the mind, movement reduces stress hormones and increases endorphins — the body's natural pain relievers.

Movement also helps rebuild strength and coordination after injury. The body heals through gradual reintroduction of motion. Staying completely still can lead to tightness, weakness, and slower recovery, while safe, structured movement prevents these setbacks.

How to Heal Through Movement

1. Start Light and Slow
Choose low-impact activities that do not cause pain.
Move gently to warm the muscles and loosen tight areas.

2. Focus on Controlled Motion
Avoid fast or explosive actions.
Smooth, slow movement activates stabilizing muscles and prevents irritation.

3. Listen to Your Body
Mild discomfort is normal, sharp pain is not.
Stop or modify movements that feel unsafe.

4. Be Consistent
Short, daily sessions are more effective than occasional long sessions.
Healing is gradual and requires regular practice.

5. Combine Motion With Breathing
Deep, calm breathing increases oxygen flow and reduces tension.

Examples of Healing Through Movement

1. Walking
One of the best low-impact ways to restore circulation.

- Helps reduce stiffness
- Improves joint mobility
- Relaxes the mind

Start with 5–10 minutes and increase gradually.

2. Gentle Stretching

Helps ease tension and improve flexibility. Examples:

- Neck stretches
- Hamstring stretch
- Chest stretch
- Hip-opening stretches

Hold each stretch lightly for 10–20 seconds.

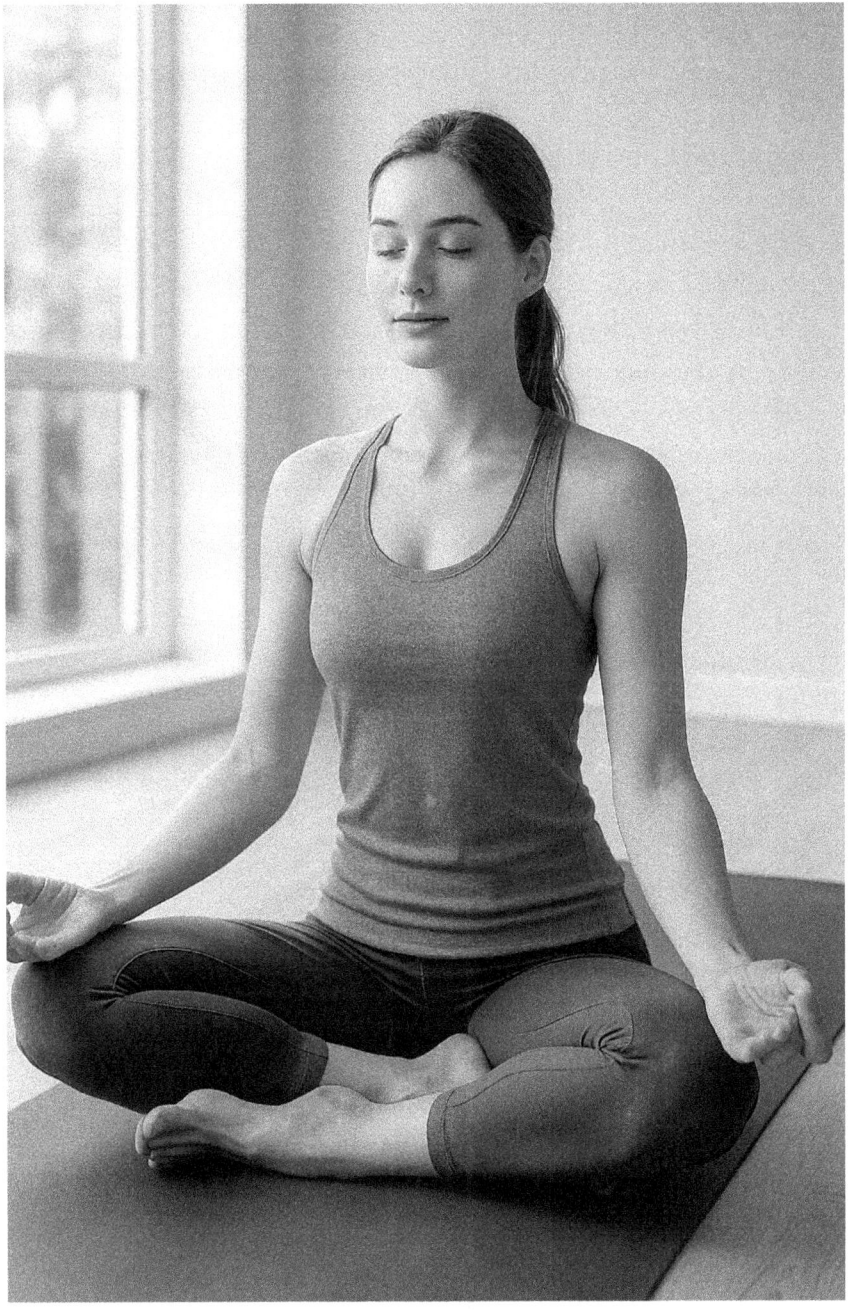

3. Yoga & Mobility Flow

Slow, controlled poses stretch tight muscles and strengthen stabilizers.

Helpful movements include:

- Cat–cow
- Child's pose
- Downward dog
- Hip mobility circles

Yoga improves both physical healing and mental relaxation.

4. Swimming or Water Movement

The water supports body weight, reducing strain on joints.

- Water walking
- Gentle swimming
- Light kicking board drills

Perfect for people with joint pain or injuries.

5. Light Cycling

Great for knees and hips because it's smooth and low-impact. Keep the resistance low and pedal slowly.

6. Foam Rolling & Self-Massage

Relieves tight muscles, improves circulation, and reduces soreness. Roll gently over:

- Quads
- Hamstrings
- Calves
- Upper back

7. Tai Chi or Slow Martial Arts

Promote balance, gentle motion, deep breathing, and mental calmness.
Perfect for emotional healing and stress reduction.

Summary

Healing through movement works by improving blood flow, reducing stiffness, restoring mobility, and supporting the body's natural repair processes. Gentle activities like walking, stretching, yoga, swimming, and mobility exercises help the body recover safely and effectively. With consistent, mindful movement, you speed up healing, reduce pain, and strengthen both the body and the mind.

10

Staying Motivated Long-Term

1. Setting Realistic Goals

Setting realistic goals is one of the most important steps in building a successful sports and fitness journey. Goals give you direction, purpose, and motivation. They help you stay focused and measure progress. However, goals must be realistic — achievable within your current fitness level, lifestyle, and timeframe. When goals are too extreme, people often become discouraged or injured. Realistic goals create steady progress, confidence, and long-term success.

How to Set Realistic Goals

1. Use the SMART Method

A realistic goal should be:

- **S**pecific
- **M**easurable
- **A**chievable
- **R**elevant
- **T**ime-bound

This structure keeps your goals clear and actionable.

2. Start From Your Current Level

Your goal should match where you are today — not where someone else is.

If you are new to running, a goal shouldn't be "run a marathon next month."

A realistic step is "jog 1 mile without stopping by the end of the month."

Understanding your starting point helps you set safe and motivating goals.

3. Break Big Goals Into Small Steps

Large goals become easier when divided into smaller milestones.
Small victories build confidence and keep you motivated.

Example:

Big goal: Lose 20 pounds

Small steps: 1–2 pounds per week through consistent exercise and nutrition.

4. Focus on Progress, Not Perfection

Realistic goals aim for steady improvement.
Progress might be slow, but small daily improvements add up to major results.

5. Be Flexible and Adjust When Needed

Life changes, injuries happen, schedules shift.
Good goals can be adjusted without guilt.
Flexibility increases long-term success.

6. Track Your Progress

Tracking shows how far you've come and keeps you accountable.
Use:

- Journals
- Fitness apps
- Photos
- Workout logs

Seeing improvement boosts motivation.

Examples of Realistic Fitness Goals

For Beginners
- Walk 20–30 minutes, 4 times a week
- Do 10 push-ups or a 30-second plank within 4 weeks
- Lose 5 pounds in one month
- Drink 6–8 cups of water daily

For Strength Training
- Increase squat weight by 10–15 pounds in 6–8 weeks
- Add 2 more reps to each set every week
- Train full body 3 days per week consistently

For Cardio & Endurance
- Jog 1 mile without stopping in 4 weeks
- Cycle 10 miles comfortably within 2 months
- Improve running time by 30 seconds over 6 weeks

For Flexibility & Mobility
- Touch your toes within 4 weeks
- Do 10 minutes of stretching after every workout

- Improve hip mobility through yoga twice a week

For Weight Loss or Muscle Gain
- Lose 1–2 pounds per week (healthy, safe rate)
- Gain 1 pound of muscle per month through strength training
- Reduce body fat by 1–2% in 6 weeks

Summary

Setting realistic goals makes fitness safe, enjoyable, and sustainable. By using the SMART method, starting from your current level, breaking goals into small steps, tracking progress, and staying flexible, you build discipline and confidence. Realistic goals lead to steady improvement — helping you stay motivated and committed to long-term health.

2. Tracking Progress

Tracking progress is one of the most effective ways to stay motivated, improve performance, and reach your health and fitness goals. When you monitor your progress, you can see what's working, make smarter adjustments, and stay committed long-term. Tracking turns your fitness journey into a measurable, rewarding process instead of guessing or hoping for results. It keeps you accountable, builds confidence, and helps you push through difficult phases.

Progress tracking is important because the body changes slowly. Without measurements, it's easy to overlook small improvements — like lifting slightly more weight, running a little faster, or feeling less tired during workouts. These small wins become clear when you track them, creating motivation and reinforcing healthy habits.

How to Track Progress

1. Keep a Workout Journal

Write down your exercises, sets, reps, weights, times, or distances. This helps you see improvement over weeks and months.

Example:

- Squat: 3×10 at 50 lbs (Week 1)
- Squat: 3×10 at 70 lbs (Week 4)
  This shows clear strength growth.

2. Track Physical Measurements

Use a tape measure or simple body measurements to track changes that aren't shown on the scale.

Track areas like:

- Waist
- Hips
- Chest
- Thighs
- Arms

This method works well for fat loss or muscle gain.

3. Take Progress Photos

Photographs show changes the scale cannot.

Take photos every 2–4 weeks in the same lighting, pose, and clothing.

Example:

Front, side, and back photos each month to see body shape changes.

4. Track Performance Improvements

Measure how your strength, speed, or endurance changes.

Examples:

- Running a mile faster
- Doing more push-ups
- Lifting heavier weights
- Holding a plank longer
- Cycling further in the same time

Performance is often a better indicator of fitness than appearance.

5. Use Apps, Wearables, or Smart Devices

Technology makes tracking easy and accurate.

Examples:

- Smart watches (steps, heart rate, distance)
- Fitness apps (workouts, calories, sleep)
- Heart rate monitors
- Pedometers

These tools show daily and weekly progress.

6. Monitor How You Feel

Track your energy, mood, stress levels, and sleep quality. These are important indicators of fitness and health.

Example:

- "Felt energized after workout"
- "Sleep improved when training 4 days a week"

Listening to your body helps prevent burnout.

7. Set Milestones and Checkpoints

Evaluate your progress every **2–4 weeks**, not every day. This prevents frustration and focuses on long-term results.

Examples of Progress Tracking for Different Goals

Strength Goal Example
- Week 1: Dead lift 100 lbs
- Week 6: Dead lift 135 lbs
  Your strength is increasing clearly.

Weight-Loss Goal Example
- Week 1: 185 lbs
- Week 4: 180 lbs
- Week 8: 178 lbs
  Slow, steady progress.

Running Goal Example
- Week 1: 1 mile = 11:30

- Week 6: 1 mile = 10:15
  Improved endurance and speed.

Flexibility Goal Example
- Week 1: Can't touch toes
- Week 5: Touch toes comfortably
  Mobility is improving.

Summary

Tracking progress in sports and fitness helps you stay motivated, measure improvement, and reach your goals faster. By using workout logs, measurements, photos, performance tests, apps, and mental check-ins, you get a clear picture of your progress. Consistent tracking turns effort into visible results, making your fitness journey more rewarding and successful.

3. Overcoming Plateaus

In sports and fitness, a **plateau** is when progress suddenly slows down or stops — even though you are still training consistently. This can happen in strength training, cardio, weight loss, flexibility, or skill development. Plateaus are frustrating but completely normal. They happen because the body adapts to routine. When your workout no longer challenges your muscles or cardiovascular system, improvement stalls. Understanding how plateaus work — and how to overcome them — is essential for long-term progress.

A plateau usually occurs for three main reasons: your body has adapted to your current workouts, your training intensity or variety is too low, or your recovery and nutrition are not supporting your goals.

The good news is that plateaus are temporary and fixable with smart changes.

How to Overcome Plateaus

1. Change Your Routine

Doing the same exercises for weeks or months causes the body to stop responding.

Switch one or more elements of your routine:

- New exercises
- New training split (upper/lower, push/pull/legs)
- Different cardio types
- New equipment

Example: Switch from regular squats to lunges, deadlifts, or goblet squats.

2. Increase Intensity (Progressive Overload)

Muscles need challenge to grow.

Increase:

- Weight
- Reps
- Sets
- Speed
- Range of motion

Example: If you've been lifting 50 lbs for weeks, increase to 55–60 lbs.

3. Adjust Training Volume

Too much or too little training can cause plateaus.
If you're overtraining, reduce volume.
If workouts are too easy, increase volume.

Example: Add one more set per exercise, or reduce total sets to allow recovery.

4. Improve Your Nutrition

The body needs fuel to grow, recover, and perform.
For strength plateaus: increase protein and calories.
For weight-loss plateaus: slightly reduce calories or increase cardio.

Example: Add an extra 20–30g of protein per day.

5. Prioritize Recovery

Not enough sleep or rest can completely stop progress.
Muscles grow *during rest*, not during the workout.

Recovery goals:

- Sleep 7–9 hours
- Take 1–2 rest days per week
- Use stretching and mobility exercises
- Try active recovery (light walking, yoga)

6. Train With Better Form

Poor technique prevents progress and increases risk of injury.
Focus on:

- Slower, controlled reps
- Full range of motion

- Correct posture

Example: A deeper squat or controlled push-up recruits more muscle.

7. Change Your Mindset

Plateaus can feel discouraging, but they are signs of growth. Use them to:

- Reevaluate your goals
- Try new styles of training
- Challenge your discipline

A plateau often means you are close to the next level.

Summary

A plateau is when progress stops because the body has adapted to your routine. Overcoming plateaus requires changes: new exercises, increased intensity, better nutrition, improved recovery, and stronger technique. With smart adjustments and patience, you break through the plateau and continue progressing safely and effectively.

4. Creating a Lifestyle of Fitness

Creating a lifestyle of fitness means turning exercise, movement, and healthy habits into a natural, sustainable part of your everyday life. Instead of viewing fitness as a temporary program or short-term challenge, it becomes a long-term commitment to feeling strong, energized, and mentally balanced. A fitness lifestyle supports not only your physical health but also your emotional and social well-being. The key is consistency — not perfection — and building habits that fit smoothly into your routine.

A fitness lifestyle starts with **small, manageable changes**. You don't need extreme workouts or strict diets. Instead, focus on daily choices that support your body. This includes regular exercise, nutritious food, hydration, sleep, and stress management. When these habits become part of your routine, fitness becomes easier and more enjoyable.

How to Create a Lifestyle of Fitness

1. Set Clear but Realistic Goals

Goals give you direction. Choose goals that motivate you, such as:

- Getting stronger
- Improving flexibility
- Losing weight
- Building endurance
- Feeling healthier

Start small, then build up. Realistic goals create confidence and long-term success.

2. Make Exercise a Routine, Not a Question

Schedule workouts like appointments.
Aim for **3–5 days per week**, even if some sessions are short.
Examples:

- Morning walk
- 20-minute home workout
- Gym session

- Evening bike ride

Consistency matters more than intensity.

3. Find Activities You Truly Enjoy

You are more likely to stick with fitness if you enjoy it. Examples:

- Group classes
- Strength training
- Yoga
- Swimming
- Sports
- Cycling

If you like it, you'll keep doing it — and that builds a lifestyle.

4. Mix Strength, Cardio & Flexibility

A balanced fitness lifestyle includes:

- **Strength training** (2–3 days/week)
- **Cardio** (3–5 days/week)
- **Stretching/mobility** (daily or after workouts)

Balance prevents boredom and reduces injury risk.

5. Maintain Healthy Eating Habits

Fitness is fueled by nutrition.
Build your lifestyle around:

- Lean proteins
- Whole grains
- Fruits and vegetables
- Healthy fats
- Proper hydration

Avoid extreme diets — focus on long-term balance.

6. Prioritize Sleep and Recovery

Rest is where the body grows stronger.
Aim for **7–9 hours** of sleep and include rest days in your routine.
Good recovery = long-term success.

7. Stay Accountable

Tracking your progress, joining classes, or training with a friend increases commitment.

Examples of accountability tools:

- Fitness apps
- Progress photos
- Workout journals
- Training partners

Accountability keeps motivation strong.

8. Build a Positive Mindset

Fitness is a journey, not a competition.
Celebrate small wins, stay patient, and remember that progress comes with time.
A positive mindset helps you stay committed even on difficult days.

Summary

Creating a lifestyle of fitness means building consistent habits — regular movement, balanced nutrition, quality sleep, and a positive mindset. By choosing enjoyable activities, setting realistic goals, and maintaining balance, fitness becomes part of daily life. This lifestyle leads to stronger health, better energy, improved confidence, and long-term well-being.

11

How Fitness Helps you overcome Depression

Depression can make the world feel heavy. It drains energy, steals motivation, and turns everyday tasks into difficult challenges. But inside the body exists a powerful, natural tool that can help fight back: **movement**. Fitness is not a cure-all, nor does it replace professional care, but it is one of the strongest, most accessible weapons against depression. When you move your body, you awaken biological, emotional, and mental systems that help lift the fog of darkness and rebuild strength from the inside out.

Fitness helps people overcome depression because it changes how the mind and body work together. Each workout, whether small or large, triggers chemical shifts that boost mood, increase self-esteem, and improve emotional resilience. Depression wants you still; movement sets you free.

1. How Movement Heals the Depressed Mind

When you engage in physical activity, your body releases **endorphins**, **dopamine**, and **serotonin** — the brain's natural antidepressants. These chemicals elevate mood, reduce anxiety, and help stabilize emotions. At the same time, exercise reduces cortisol, the stress hormone that often fuels depressive symptoms.

Movement also improves **blood flow and oxygenation** to the brain. This enhances mental clarity, reduces the feeling of being mentally "stuck," and increases overall cognitive performance. Studies show that consistent exercise can be just as effective as medication for mild to moderate depression — without harmful side effects.

But the benefits are not only chemical. Fitness encourages **routine**, **discipline**, and **positive identity**, all of which are essential for emotional healing.

Every workout is a message to yourself:
"I am healing. I am capable. I am moving forward."

Fitness does not replace professional treatment, but it is one of the most powerful tools you can use to support your recovery. Motion creates emotion — and even the smallest steps can lead you out of the darkest places.

2. The First Step: Starting Small

For someone struggling with depression, even getting out of bed can feel overwhelming. This is why the first step in fitness-based healing must be **small, achievable, and forgiving**.

Start with one of the following:

- Five minutes of walking
- Ten deep breaths and a gentle stretch
- A short yoga video
- One set of bodyweight exercises
- Walking around the block

The goal is not perfection — it is momentum. Small wins create energy. Energy creates hope. Hope creates action.

Even the lightest workout sends a message to your brain:
"I am fighting. I am alive. I am capable."

3. Real-Life Stories of Healing Through Fitness

Story 1: Walking Toward the Light

Lena, a 36-year-old teacher, felt trapped in depression after a difficult divorce. She didn't have strength for the gym, but she began walking each morning for just ten minutes. At first, she cried during the walks — but she kept going. Soon, ten minutes turned into twenty. Then an hour.

Hiking trails replaced city streets. Sunlight replaced darkness. Her thoughts became clearer with each step.

Walking didn't erase her problems, but it gave her the power to face them again.

Story 2: Strength Training That Rebuilt a Broken Spirit

Mike, 29, felt worthless after losing his job. Depression made him feel weak inside and out. A friend convinced him to join a gym. Mike began with light dumbbells — nothing heavy, nothing fast. After a month, he noticed he could lift more weight. His muscles grew, but so did his confidence.

Strength training gave him proof that he could improve and control something in his life.

One day he looked in the mirror and realized:

He wasn't just lifting weights — he was lifting himself out of despair.

Story 3: Yoga as a Quiet Rescue

Hannah suffered from anxiety and depression so deeply that her thoughts felt like storms. A gentle yoga class changed everything. Learning to control her breath calmed the storms inside her mind. The stretching relieved tension in her body. The peaceful environment felt safe.

Yoga gave her the quiet she needed to heal.

4. Best Types of Fitness for Fighting Depression

Walking or Hiking
One of the most effective mood boosters.
Benefits: clears the mind, reduces stress hormones, improves sleep.

Strength Training
Builds confidence, structure, and power.
Benefits: increases self-esteem and supports long-term mood stability.

Yoga or Pilates
Calms the nervous system and improves emotional control.
Benefits: reduces anxiety and improves mindfulness.

Cycling or Running
Raises heart rate and releases strong levels of endorphins.
Benefits: improves cardiovascular health and reduces fatigue.

Group Fitness or Sports
Provides community, motivation, and belonging.
Benefits: reduces isolation, enhances confidence.

5. How Fitness Builds Hope and Identity

Depression often tells people that they are weak, hopeless, or broken. Fitness proves the opposite.

Every workout, no matter how small, builds the following:

- **Confidence**

You see progress over time.

- **Purpose**

You have a reason to get up and move.

- **Structure**

Routines help stabilize emotions.

- **Social Connection**

Gyms, classes, and outdoor groups combat loneliness.

- **Self-Control**

You learn that you can shape your life through action.

- **Identity**

"I am someone who shows up for myself."

This psychological shift is one of the most powerful tools for overcoming depression.

6. A Simple Weekly Plan for Healing Through Movement

Day 1: 20-minute walk + light stretching
Day 2: Strength training (20–30 minutes)
Day 3: Gentle yoga (15–20 minutes)
Day 4: Walk in nature or a local park
Day 5: Strength or resistance bands
Day 6: Choose an enjoyable activity (dance, biking, swimming)
Day 7: Rest, relax, breathe

The plan is flexible. The only rule is: **move every day**, even if it's just a few minutes.

7. When Fitness Becomes Healing

Over time, fitness stops feeling like effort and starts feeling like therapy. Your body becomes stronger, your mind becomes clearer, and your spirit becomes lighter. Depression loses its grip as movement builds momentum, direction, and identity.

Fitness gives you moments of joy, moments of pride, moments of silence, and moments of power. When you combine these moments, you create a pathway out of darkness.

Final Message: You Are Stronger Than You Think

Depression tells you to be still.
Movement tells you to rise.

Every stretch, every breath, every walk becomes a step toward healing.

Fitness is not about perfection — it is about progress.

It is about rediscovering your strength, rebuilding your hope, and remembering that your story is not finished.

You do not need to overcome depression all at once.

You only need to take the next small step.

Your body will help your mind — and your mind will help your life.

You are not alone.

You are not broken.

You are capable of rising again.

And every moment of movement is proof.

You don't need extreme workouts to fight depression.

You only need movement — gentle, consistent, and forgiving.

Every walk, every stretch, every push-up tells your brain:

"I am healing. I am getting stronger."

Real Story: How One Person Won the Battle Against Depression

For most of his adult life, David was known as the friendly coworker, the dependable friend, the one who always helped others smile. What no one saw was the storm happening inside him. At 34, after a painful breakup and losing a job he had held for nearly a decade, depression hit him harder than anything before. He stopped leaving the house. Stopped answering messages. Days blended into nights, and even simple tasks — eating, showering, getting out of bed — felt impossible.

One afternoon, after weeks of isolation, David's sister visited him. She didn't lecture or push him. She just sat with him and said, "Let's walk for five minutes. If you want to stop, we stop." He didn't want to go, but something in her gentle tone made him nod.

They walked to the end of the street. David's legs felt heavy, his chest tight. But when they reached the corner, he realized — just for a moment — he could breathe a little deeper. That five-minute walk became the first tiny spark of light in a very dark tunnel.

The next day, he walked alone. Five minutes turned into eight. Then ten. The world outside slowly felt less threatening. He began noticing things he hadn't seen in months — sunlight warming his face, birds singing on rooftops, neighbors waving hello. Those walks didn't cure his depression overnight, but they interrupted the cycle of stillness and rumination that kept him trapped.

A few weeks later, David joined a small community fitness program at the local park. The first day, he could barely do the warm-up. He felt embarrassed and almost quit. But an older man in the group smiled and said, "Hey, you showed up. That's the hardest part." For the first time in months, David felt seen — not as a broken person, but as someone trying.

Slowly, exercise became his anchor.
• Strength training gave him a sense of power again.
• Running cleared his mind of negative thoughts.
• Group fitness gave him support and connection.

He wasn't fighting alone anymore.

As the months passed, something changed inside him. He started sleeping better. His appetite returned. The constant heaviness in his chest loosened. And little victories — lifting a heavier weight, jogging a little farther, laughing with others — reminded him he was capable.

One evening, after finishing a run longer than he ever imagined possible, David sat on a bench overlooking the park. He felt tired, sweating, but alive in a way he hadn't felt in years. He realized that fitness hadn't just strengthened his body — it had rebuilt his identity, his confidence, and his hope.

Depression still whispered occasionally, but he no longer believed its lies.

He had proof of his strength — in every step he walked, every weight he lifted, every breath he took outdoors.

David didn't "snap out" of depression.

He *walked out* of it, one small step at a time — until the steps became strides, and the strides became a new life.

And whenever someone asks him how he survived, he simply says:

"Motion saved me. Movement gave me back the person I thought I lost."

12

Special Training for Different Ages

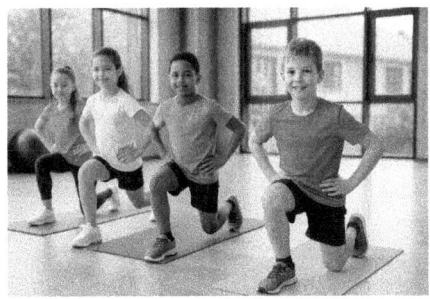

1. Kids & Teen Fitness

Kids and teens need fitness just as much as adults — not for weight loss or extreme training, but for developing strong bodies, healthy habits, emotional stability, and lifelong confidence. **Kids & Teen Fitness** refers to age-appropriate physical activity that builds strength, coordination, endurance, balance, and overall well-being. The goal is not intense workouts or professional athletics — it is movement that supports growth, fun, and healthy development.

During childhood and teenage years, the body is growing rapidly. Muscles, bones, nerves, and hormones all change quickly. Regular physical activity helps these systems grow strong and balanced. Fitness also improves heart health, builds healthy bones, supports brain development, and reduces stress. Kids who stay active are more confident, sleep better, concentrate better in school, and develop stronger emotional resilience.

However, training for kids and teens must be **safe, enjoyable, and age-appropriate**. Overtraining or using adult-level workouts can harm developing bones, joints, and muscles. The best approach is making fitness fun, varied, and skill-based.

How Kids & Teens Should Train (Best Methods)

1. Focus on Fun, Not Pressure

Children and teens are more likely to stay active when the activity is enjoyable.

- Games
- Sports
- Team activities
- Outdoor play

Fun creates long-term fitness habits.

2. Build Basic Movement Skills

Before heavy training, kids need fundamental skills:

- Running
- Jumping
- Throwing
- Catching
- Balancing

- Climbing

  These build coordination and athletic foundation.

3. Strength Training is Safe — When Done Correctly

Kids can safely do strength training using:

- Bodyweight exercises
- Light resistance bands
- Medicine balls
- Simple machines with low weight
- Proper technique

Examples:

- Squats
- Lunges
- Push-ups
- Planks
- Step-ups
- Wall sits

Heavy barbells or max lifts should be avoided until late teens unless guided by a certified coach.

4. Cardio Should Be Natural and Playful

Kids don't need long-distance running programs. Use fun, short activities such as:

- Tag
- Biking
- Swimming
- Jump rope
- Sports like soccer, basketball, or tennis

This builds stamina without boredom.

5. Encourage Flexibility & Mobility

Growing bodies need stretching to reduce tightness and prevent injury.

- Light yoga
- Dynamic stretching
- Gentle post-workout stretches

6. Limit Sedentary Time

Too much screen time affects posture, mood, and energy. Encourage movement every day.

7. Teach Healthy Habits

Kids should learn:

- Good posture
- Safe lifting technique
- The importance of hydration

- Balanced meals
- Rest and sleep

This builds lifelong responsibility.

8. Avoid Overtraining & Competition Pressure

Kids develop best when they enjoy the process, not when pushed too hard.
Watch for signs of:

- Excess fatigue
- Pain
- Stress
- Anxiety

Safety and enjoyment come first.

Summary

Kids & Teen Fitness is about building healthy habits, strong bodies, and positive attitudes toward movement. The best training includes fun activities, basic skill development, light strength training, playful cardio, stretching, and good lifestyle habits. When fitness is enjoyable, safe, and balanced, children and teens grow into healthier, more confident adults with lifelong love for physical activity.

2. Adults 20–45

Adults aged **20–45** are in a uniquely powerful stage of life for fitness. The body is strong, flexible, and capable of building muscle, improving endurance, and enhancing overall performance. Training during these years creates long-lasting health benefits, supports mental well-being, and prevents future health problems. The best training for adults in this age range balances **strength, cardio, mobility, and recovery** — giving the body exactly what it needs to stay strong and functional.

This age group often faces busy schedules, stress, and lifestyle pressure. Proper training helps maintain energy, manage weight, increase confidence, and support longevity. The right fitness plan strengthens both the body and the mind.

Why Training is Important for Ages 20-45

1. Peak Muscle-Building Years

Adults 20–45 can build muscle more easily than older adults due to optimal hormone levels.
Strength training now creates:

- Stronger bones
- Higher metabolism
- Injury prevention
- Better posture

Building muscle early protects you later in life.

2. Heart Health & Metabolism

Cardio training improves:

- Blood pressure

- Heart function
- Lung capacity
- Fat burning

This age range is the best time to build lifelong cardiovascular health.

3. Stress Reduction & Mental Health

Fitness reduces anxiety, depression, anger, and mental fatigue. Adults gain:

- Better focus
- Improved sleep
- Emotional balance
- More confidence

This supports work, relationships, and daily life.

4. Weight Control & Body Composition

Muscle mass naturally declines after age 30.
Training helps maintain or increase muscle, keeping:

- Body fat lower
- Weight stable
- Energy higher

This prevents long-term metabolic issues.

5. Long-Term Injury Prevention

Strong muscles and mobile joints reduce the risk of injuries from:

- Work
- Daily tasks
- Sports
- Aging

Training in this age group builds the foundation for healthy aging.

How Adults (20–45) Should Train

The ideal fitness routine includes **4 key components**:

1. Strength Training (2–4 times per week)

Strength work is the most important part of training for adults.
Benefits: muscle growth, strong joints, faster metabolism, better posture.
Best exercises:

- Squats
- Deadlifts
- Bench press or push-ups
- Rows
- Lunges
- Shoulder press
- Core exercises (planks, leg raises)

Equipment options: dumbbells, barbells, resistance bands, machines, bodyweight.

2. Cardiovascular Training (2–4 times per week)

Cardio keeps your heart and lungs strong.
Types of cardio:

- Running or jogging
- Cycling
- Swimming
- Rowing
- Brisk walking
- HIIT (High-Intensity Interval Training)

Goal: 150–300 minutes of moderate cardio per week or 75 minutes of intense cardio.

3. Mobility & Flexibility (daily or after workouts)

Mobility keeps your body pain-free and flexible.
Examples:

- Stretching
- Yoga
- Foam rolling
- Hip mobility drills
- Shoulder mobility exercises

This improves posture, prevents injury, and keeps joints healthy.

4. Recovery & Lifestyle Habits

Adults must balance fitness with life demands.
Key components:

- 7–9 hours of sleep
- Hydration
- Balanced meals
- Rest days
- Stress management

Recovery allows the body to grow stronger.

Sample Weekly Training for Adults (20–45)

Monday: Strength Training (Full Body)
Tuesday: Cardio (Jogging, cycling, or HIIT)
Wednesday: Light activity + Stretching
Thursday: Strength Training
Friday: Cardio or Sport
Saturday: Mobility, yoga, or active recovery
Sunday: Rest

Summary

For adults aged 20–45, the best training combines **strength, cardio, mobility, and recovery**. This approach maximizes muscle growth, supports heart health, reduces stress, improves confidence, and builds long-term resilience. Training in these prime years builds the foundation for a healthier, stronger life — now and for decades ahead.

3. Seniors 50+

Fitness for adults aged **50 and older** is essential for maintaining independence, preventing injuries, and improving quality of life. At this stage, the goal of training is not extreme intensity — it is **strength, mobility, balance, joint health, and overall functional fitness**. The right exercise plan helps seniors move with confidence, reduce pain, maintain energy, and protect the body from age-related decline. With safe, consistent training, people over 50 can feel healthier and stronger than ever.

As the body ages, muscle mass naturally decreases, joints become stiffer, and balance may weaken. The best training for seniors targets these areas with gentle, smart, and purposeful exercises. Even beginners can see major improvements within a few weeks.

Why Training Is Important for Seniors 50+

1. Maintain Muscle & Strength

After age 50, muscle loss speeds up (sarcopenia). Strength training slows or reverses this, helping with:

- Daily tasks (lifting, walking, stairs)
- Independence
- Posture
- Joint protection

2. Improve Balance & Prevent Falls

Falls are a major risk for older adults. Balance training strengthens stabilizing muscles and coordination.

3. Reduce Joint Pain

Movement increases lubrication in the joints and reduces stiffness. Low-impact exercise helps with arthritis and back pain.

4. Boost Heart & Lung Health

Cardio keeps the heart strong, improves circulation, and increases stamina.

5. Improve Mood, Memory & Energy

Exercise boosts blood flow to the brain and reduces stress hormones. Fitness supports emotional health and reduces anxiety.

6. Protect Bone Health

Weight-bearing exercise helps prevent osteoporosis.

Best Training Types for Seniors 50+

1. Strength Training (2–3 times per week)

Safe and gentle strength training is the foundation of senior fitness.
Best exercises:

- Bodyweight squats or chair squats
- Resistance band rows
- Light dumbbell exercises
- Wall push-ups or incline push-ups
- Step-ups
- Glute bridges
- Core exercises (bird-dog, planks, dead bug)

Benefits: Stronger muscles, better balance, joint support, improved metabolism.

2. Low-Impact Cardio (3–5 days per week)

Low-impact cardio is safe for joints and great for heart health.
Best options:

- Walking
- Cycling (indoor or outdoor)
- Swimming or water aerobics
- Elliptical machines
- Light hiking

Goal: 20–40 minutes per session.

3. Flexibility & Mobility (daily)

Stretching helps reduce stiffness and improve joint movement.
Great choices:

- Gentle yoga
- Tai Chi
- Light stretching
- Shoulder mobility
- Hip and back stretches

This improves posture, reduces pain, and increases range of motion.

4. Balance Training (3+ days per week)

Balance exercises reduce fall risk and improve stability.
Examples:

- Standing on one leg
- Heel-to-toe walking
- Side leg lifts
- Step taps
- Slow-paced agility drills

Even 5 minutes a day helps a lot.

5. Functional Training

Movements that mimic real-life activities.
Examples:

- Carrying light weights (grocery bags simulation)
- Hip hinges (safe bending)
- Sit-to-stand exercises
- Reaching and rotation exercises

This keeps daily life easier and safer.

Safety Tips for Seniors 50+

- Warm up gently before exercise
- Start slow and progress gradually
- Use light weights or resistance bands
- Avoid high-impact movements or heavy lifting without guidance
- Stop if experiencing sharp pain or dizziness

- Stay hydrated
- Consult a doctor if you have medical conditions

Summary

The best training for seniors 50+ focuses on **strength, balance, mobility, flexibility, and low-impact cardio**. These exercises protect joints, prevent injuries, increase independence, and improve energy and mood. With consistent, safe, and enjoyable training, adults over 50 can stay strong, active, and healthy for many years.

4. Safe Sports for All Ages

Safe sports for all ages refers to physical activities that can be done safely by children, teens, adults, and seniors — without high risk of injury, stress, or overexertion. These sports focus on **low-impact movement, proper technique, age-appropriate intensity, and long-term enjoyment**. The goal is to keep everyone active, healthy, and confident, regardless of age or fitness level. Safe sports help improve heart health, muscle strength, balance, mobility, and mental well-being while reducing the chance of injury.

Safety in sport means choosing the right activities, warming up properly, using correct equipment, avoiding overtraining, and adjusting exercises to match each person's physical ability. With the right approach, people from **kids to seniors 70+** can enjoy movement comfortably and effectively.

How to Practice Safe Sports at Any Age

1. Choose Low-Impact Activities

Low-impact sports reduce stress on joints and muscles.

Examples by Age Group:
Kids & Teens:

- Swimming
- Biking
- Soccer (light, recreational)
- Dance
- Basketball (non-competitive)

Adults:

- Walking or hiking
- Cycling
- Swimming
- Rowing
- Fitness classes (moderate intensity)

Seniors 50+:

- Walking
- Water aerobics
- Tai Chi
- Light cycling
- Gentle yoga

These activities support heart health and endurance without excessive strain.

2. Use Proper Technique

Correct form protects the body and improves performance.

Tips:
- Learn basics before increasing intensity
- Use lighter weights until technique is perfect
- Avoid rushing or forcing movements
- Ask a coach or trainer for help if needed

Proper technique makes sport safer for every age.

3. Adjust Intensity to Fitness Level

The same sport can be safe for all ages if intensity is appropriate.

Examples:
- Kids: run in short bursts, play games
- Adults: steady jogging, cycling at moderate speed
- Seniors: brisk walking or gentle swimming

Modify pace, duration, or resistance to match ability.

4. Warm Up & Cool Down

Warm-ups prepare the body and reduce injury risk. Cool-downs relax muscles and improve recovery.

Simple Warm-Up Examples:
- Light walking
- Arm circles
- Leg swings

- Slow stretching

Warm-ups are essential at any age.

5. Use the Right Equipment

Safe sports require proper shoes, protective gear, and comfortable clothing.

Examples:
- Helmets for biking
- Supportive shoes for walking or running
- Water shoes for pool workouts
- Knee or wrist supports if needed for seniors

Good equipment prevents injuries.

6. Listen to Your Body

If something hurts, stop.
Pain, dizziness, or heavy fatigue are warning signs.

Safe rule for all ages:
- Slight discomfort = okay
- Sharp pain = stop immediately

Adjust training as needed.

7. *Stay Hydrated & Rest*

Hydration and rest keep performance strong and prevent overexertion.

Guidelines:
- Drink water before, during, after activity
- Take rest days
- Sleep 7–9 hours for recovery

Rest is key to long-term safety.

Examples of Safe Sports for All Ages

1. Walking
- Best all-age activity
- Improves heart health, reduces stress, strengthens legs

2. Swimming / Water Aerobics
- Gentle on joints
- Builds endurance and strength
- Great for kids, adults, seniors

3. Cycling
- Low-impact
- Builds leg strength and stamina
- Safe when done on flat paths

4. Yoga & Stretching
- Improves flexibility, balance, and mental health
- Can be adapted from beginner to advanced

5. Light Strength Training
- Safe with proper form
- Improves bone and muscle health
- Use bodyweight or light resistance

Summary

Safe sports for all ages combine low-impact movement, proper technique, age-appropriate intensity, and good equipment. Activities like walking, swimming, yoga, and cycling are safe and effective for children, adults, and seniors. With warm-ups, hydration, and mindful progress, anyone can enjoy fitness safely and build lifelong health

13

Conclusion: Living the Strong Life

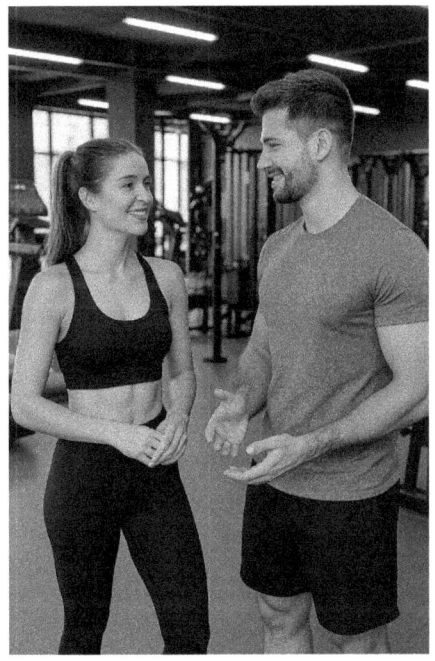

Living a strong, healthy life is not just about having a fit body — it is about creating harmony between **physical strength**, **mental clarity**, and **emotional resilience**. Fitness and sports give you the tools to build a powerful, capable body while also shaping a focused and confident mind. When you commit to movement, you improve every part of your life: your energy, mood, discipline, creativity, and sense of purpose.

— CONCLUSION: LIVING THE STRONG LIFE

Sports strengthen the **body** by improving muscle tone, endurance, heart health, mobility, and overall physical power. Strength training builds solid muscles and bones. Cardio strengthens the heart and lungs. Flexibility work keeps you agile and pain-free. These benefits help you move easier, breathe better, and stay active for years to come.

At the same time, sports strengthen the **mind**. Physical activity releases endorphins, reduces stress hormones, sharpens focus, improves memory, and boosts confidence. It teaches discipline, patience, and mental toughness. Whether it's running, swimming, lifting weights, or practicing yoga, every workout strengthens your mindset as much as your muscles.

The combination of body and mind fitness leads to a life of balance, resilience, and self-belief. Here are examples of how fitness supports your whole life: **How Fitness Helps the Body & Mind (With Examples)**

1. **Strength Training for Physical Power**
   - Builds strong muscles and bones
   - Improves posture and daily movement
   - Increases confidence and determination

2. **Cardio for Heart & Mood Health**
   - Running or cycling boosts heart health
   - Reduces anxiety and depression
   - Improves endurance in both physical and mental tasks

3. **Flexibility & Mobility for Pain-Free Living**
   - Yoga or stretching reduces stiffness
   - Prevents injury
   - Calms the mind and reduces stress

4. Sports for Social & Emotional Strength
- Team sports build communication and community
- Improve emotional resilience
- Create joy, fun, and motivation

5. Recovery & Balance for Long-Term Well-Being
- Rest days restore energy
- Sleep strengthens immune function and memory
- Relaxation practices maintain mental balance

Why This Matters

When fitness becomes part of your lifestyle, you build a body that supports your goals and a mind that can overcome challenges. You become more capable, confident, focused, and emotionally steady. You gain the ability to handle pressure, stay positive, and live with strength and intention.

Fitness does not require perfection — only consistency. Small steps done daily create lifelong transformation. Every walk, every stretch, every workout builds a healthier future.

Living the Strong Life

Living the strong life means choosing habits that protect your health, elevate your mind, and strengthen your spirit. It means committing to movement, respecting your body, and embracing challenges as opportunities to grow. Strength is not just physical — it is the courage to take care of yourself, the discipline to stay consistent, and the belief that you deserve a powerful, healthy life.

No matter your age, background, or fitness level, you can begin today.

Move your body. Train your mind. Build your life.

This is the path to living strong — now and for the rest of your life.

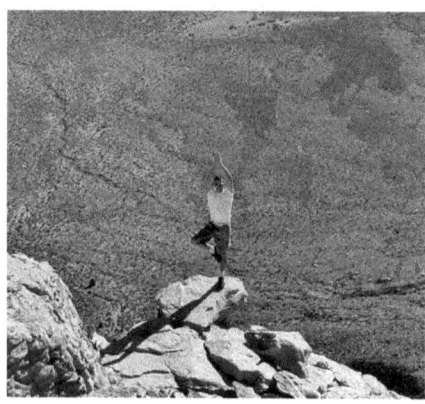

HEALTH AND LONGEST LIFE FOR YOU!!!

TIM KORSA, who has been living an active lifestyle for over 50 years, has competed in many different sports like Triathlon, Boxing and Kickboxing, competed in many different countries, Run Boston Marathon, Chicago Sun Time Triathlon and others. Have Fitness Nutrition Diploma. Wish to People Health and be stronger.

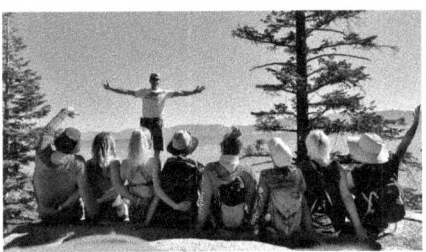

www.ingramcontent.com/pod-product-compliance
Lightning Source LLC
Chambersburg PA
CBHW070628030426
42337CB00020B/3954